DR. EARL MINDELL'S GUIDE TO

HEALING WITH
CBD

Other Books by the Author

The Happiness Effect

What You Must Know About Allergy Relief
with Pamela Wartian Smith, MD, MPH

What You Must Know About Homeopathic Remedies

Healing With Hemp CBD Oil

DR. EARL MINDELL'S GUIDE TO

HEALING WITH
CBD

How to Maximize the Healing Power of CBD for Your Health

EARL MINDELL, RPH, MH, PHD

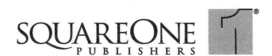

SQUAREONE
PUBLISHERS

The information and advice contained in this book are based upon the research and the personal and professional experiences of the authors. They are not intended as a substitute for consulting with a health care professional. The publisher and author are not responsible for any adverse effects or consequences resulting from the use of any of the suggestions, preparations, or procedures discussed in this book. All matters pertaining to your physical health should be supervised by a health care professional. It is a sign of wisdom, not cowardice, to seek a second or third opinion.

EDITOR: Erica Shur
COVER & INTERIOR DESIGNER: Gary A. Rosenberg

Square One Publishers

115 Herricks Road
Garden City Park, NY 11040
(516) 535-2010 • (877) 900-BOOK
www.squareonepublishers.com

Library of Congress Cataloging-in-Publication Data
Names: Mindell, Earl, author.
Title: Dr. Earl Mindell's guide to healing with CBD : how to maximize the healing power of CBD for your health / Earl Mindell, RPh, MH, PhD. Description: Garden City Park, NY : Square One Publishers, [2021] | Includes bibliographical references and index. | Summary: "The guide is divided into two parts. Part One is devoted to making you a smart consumer who knows how to buy, use, and store CBD oil-based products. Part Two provides a listing of specific health disorders and how CBD oil can be used to relieve them. Each entry includes an explanation of the problem, its most common symptoms, its triggers, and its standard conventional treatment and side effects, if any. The entry concludes with a discussion of how you can use CBD oil to improve your health"— Provided by publisher.
Identifiers: LCCN 2021031331 (print) | LCCN 2021031332 (ebook) | ISBN 9780757005213 (paperback) | ISBN 9780757055218 (ebook)
Subjects: LCSH: Cannabis--Therapeutic use. | Cannabinoids--Therapeutic use.
Classification: LCC RM666.C266 M563 2021 (print) | LCC RM666.C266 (ebook) | DDC 615.7/827--dc23
LC record available at https://lccn.loc.gov/2021031331
LC ebook record available at https://lccn.loc.gov/2021031332

Printed in the United States of America

10   9   8   7   6   5   4   3   2   1

Contents

Introduction, 1

A Buyer's Guide to CBD, 3

An Alphabetical Guide to Using CBD, 25

Addiction, Opiate, 25

ADHD, 27

Age-Related Macular
Degeneration, 28

Alzheimer's Disease, 30

AMD, 33

Anxiety Disorders, 33

Appetite Loss, 35

Arthritis, 37

Attention Deficit
Hyperactivity , 39

Disorder, 39

Blood Clots, 42

Cancer, 45

Cardiovascular Disease, 47

Chemotherapy, Side
Effects, 48

Colitis, Ulcerative, 48

Crohn's Disease, 48

Depression, 50

Dermatitis, Atopic, 52

Eczema, 53

Epilepsy, 56

Eye Disorders, 59

Fibromyalgia, 59

FM, 61

Glaucoma, 61

Headache, 63

Heart Disease, 66

High Blood Pressure, 68

Inflammation, 71

Insomnia, 74

Irritable Bowel Syndrome, 77

Macular Degeneration, 80

Menopause, 80

Migraine Headache, 80

MS, 81

Multiple Sclerosis, 81

Nausea And Vomiting, 85

Opiate Addiction, 87

Panic Attack, 87

PMS, 87

Post Traumatic Stress Disorder, 87

Premenstrual Syndrome, 87

Schizophrenia, 90

Skin Conditions, 92

Sleep Disorders, 92

Thrombosis, 92

Thyroid Disorder, 93

Ulcerative Colitis, 93

Resources, 97

About the Author, 99

Index, 100

Introduction

Imagine that researchers had found a naturally occurring substance that could effectively overcome dozens of health disorders without any serious side effects. Now imagine that the plant in which this substance was found had been banned in this country because, as a commercially grown crop, it threatened other competing "cash" crops. As new studies showed its many medical benefits, our laws continued to prevent farmers from planting an easy-to-grow crop that requires few, if any, pesticides or herbicides. If you think that sounds so crazy that it couldn't be true, think again. For the last seventy years, the Federal government has prohibited farmers from commercially growing the hemp plant. In doing so, it has effectively prevented American companies from making available extracts with CBD—the very compound that science has found to be an amazing and versatile healer.

As it turns out, hemp is a relative of marijuana. Both are *cannabis* plants, as are many other plants. However, while marijuana is high in THC, the chemical compound that accounts for marijuana's psychoactive effects, hemp contains too little of this chemical to get anyone high. On the other hand, while most available marijuana contains a relatively low level of the healing compound CBD, hemp is high in CBD—which has no psychoactive effects and is non-toxicating. Yet as you will discover in the chapters that follow, for decades, the hemp plant has been outlawed along with marijuana because the government has falsely classified it as a dangerous Schedule 1 drug. And while more and more states are legalizing the growth and sale of marijuana, hemp is still not permitted to be grown as a commercial crop.

As a registered pharmacist, I have witnessed the amazing growth of pharmaceutical companies over the years. I have also seen too many of these companies produce drugs that may relieve specific symptoms but come with dangerous side effects. I have always looked for natural products that can provide the same relief without the risk of side effects. That is not to say that pharmaceutical companies don't produce life-saving drugs, because they do.

However, nature has provided us with many alternative solutions that work well. Over the years, as I read more about the many benefits of hemp oil extracts and CBD, I discovered that hemp's classification as a Schedule 1 drug made no sense in light of the available scientific research. I needed to know more.

Dr. Earl Mindell's Guide to Healing with CBD is the result of my investigation into this important supplement. The guide is divided into two parts. Part One is devoted to making you a smart consumer, who knows how to buy, use, and store CBD oil-based products.

Part Two provides a listing of specific health disorders and how CBD can be used to relieve them. Each entry includes an explanation of the problem, its most common symptoms, its causes, and its standard conventional treatment and side effects, if any. The entry concludes with a discussion of how you can use CBD to improve your health.

At the end of the book, a resource section guides you to the organizations and websites that can assist you in learning more about CBD.

The information presented in this guide is not meant to replace the medical advice given to you by your physician. It is designed to provide the facts you need to know to make informed decisions about your health. If in reading this guide you find a treatment that is of interest to you, do not be afraid to discuss it with your doctor. You can play an important role in your own health or healing process.

A Buyer's Guide to CBD

As an informed consumer, it is important to know the differences between the many varieties of CBD extracts and the numerous products and delivery systems that are available on the market. CBD is produced in the US and under federal law CBD oils can be legally imported into the United Sates. Thus, with the growing availability of CBD extracts, the information out there can be very confusing when it comes to determining which CBD preparations are the best—and perhaps most effective. This chapter will explain some of the confusing terms used to describe these products. We will then discuss some of the common products found on the shelves, what to look for on the labels, and in some cases, what ingredients to avoid. And just as important, you will learn how to properly store all these items.

WHAT IS CBD OIL?

If you do any research online, it is likely you will see products referred to as CBD oil, CBD extracts, or CBD cannabidiol oil. You may also see contradictory statements as to what makes them different from one another. It can all be very confusing, so let's start with a quick refresher course. The two best-know members of the Cannabis family are marijuana and hemp. They grow as plants sprouting stalks, leaves and flowers. Each of these plants contains THC and CBD. While the marijuana variety contains more THC, from 5 to 20 percent, hemp plants contain only a fraction of this amount, not exceeding the legal limit of 0.3 percent THC (on a dry weight basis). Normally all commercially available CBD products come from the agricultural hemp plant.

Oil can be extracted from any and all parts of the cannabis plant. This includes its stalk, leaves, flowers, seeds, roots, and/ or branches. The terms "CBD oil," and "CBD extracts" are often interchanged, and often fail to clearly communicate to consumers exactly what is in the bottle being sold. The lack of standardization in this new language is expected and is due to the ambiguity surrounding the regulatory future of these products. The most important rule is not to confuse hemp seed oil with hemp extracts when you are looking for CBD.

CBD oil extracts do contain CBD and THC. Depending on the environmental conditions and plant genetics used to make the extract, this results in products with a wide variation in ratios of CBD to THC, with wide ranging legal implications. The finished CBD product may therefore qualify as either a medical marijuana or agricultural product that contains naturally occurring CBD.

The easiest way to tell the difference between hemp seed oil and hemp CBD is to make absolutely sure that the Supplement facts panel on the back of the bottle reads "CBD oil (aerial plant parts)." There should be a total milligram amount of hemp oil on the first line with the second line below it listing the total cannabidiol in milligrams of CBD per serving. Another factor to consider when choosing a CBD oil is its refinement and concentration.

Raw Hemp CBD Oil

Raw hemp CBD oil extract is a powerful full spectrum hemp superfood. The majority of cannabinoids in raw hemp oil extracts is comprised of cannabidiolic acid, or CBDA. CBDA is the acidic precursor of CBD, which is naturally produced in the plant and contains many beneficial properties distinct from CBD. This type of CBD oil can be used as an anti-inflammatory for systemic inflammation. Some of the issues raw CBD oil may affect are nausea, pain, acute orthopedic injuries, exercise-induced muscle soreness, rheumatoid arthritis, cancer cell migration, and autoimmune conditions. Since this type of oil is the least refined, it has less of a blood-brain barrier penetration and thus is least likely to cause any effects to the central nervous system (CNS) such as somnolence.

Decarboxylated CBD Oil

When raw CBD oil is gently heated in a process known as decarboxylation, the natural CBDA content in the extract is converted to activated CBD. The carboxylic acid group simply breaks off changing the structure and function of CBDA to fully activated CBD. Although many compounds existing in nature activate the endocannabinoid system, CBD is exclusively a byproduct of the decarboxylation of CBDA, meaning the near exclusive source of CBD in nature comes from heating or exposure to light in order to potentiate the chemical conversion of CBDA into activated CBD.

Hemp extracts made from certified agricultural are considered full-spectrum because they contain a wide range of natural phytocannabinoids, such as CBD, CBG, CBN, CBC, and traces of other cannabinoids in addition to the other natural cofactors, including plant sterols, terpenes, chlorophyll, and all eight isomers of naturally occurring vitamin E. When activated, CBD crosses the blood-brain barrier and is reported to have profound effects in supporting nervous system health, anxiety, stress, depression, sleep, increasing insulin sensitivity, and may be used as a peripheral immunomodulator or anti-inflammatory.

The dosing strategy for decarboxylated CBD Oil is always to start low (~ 2 mg of CBD) and titrate up (~ 15 mg of CBD) as needed. A protocol has been circulating for three years in the natural remedies community that recommends starting with a CBD product that delivers either 2 mg or 3 mg per serving and slowly increasing the dosage of CBD to 15 mg per day over several weeks for people who are very sick, or a few days for those with more well-balanced endocannabinoid tone. The goal is to titrate the dose to minimize secondary effects like somnolence.

Optimizing and fine-tuning our endocannabinoid system may be the ultimate self-hacking modality to truly promote healing and restore balance. You may want to combine some raw CBDA rich full spectrum extract with some activated CBD oil extract for additional full plant, broad spectrum synergy and support.

Gold Formula CBD Oil

Gold extracts are standardized—similar to other herbal extracts—where the plant material is distilled in a solvent-free process, concentrating CBD, other cannabinoids, fatty acids, terpenes, and naturally-occurring vitamin E. In fact, it takes approximately 10 kilograms of decarboxylated CBD oil extract to yield approximately 3 kilograms of gold concentrated CBD oil extract.

Concentrated CBD oil combined with lipid excipients like extra virgin olive oil have a faster onset of use because they contain more fats and fatty acids that increase the bioavailability of the fat-loving cannabinoid CBD by three-fold. Gold extracts also have the highest concentration and amount of the full range of phytocannabinoids available in hemp, including ten times more of the micro-dosage of natural THC than the starting raw hemp extract itself. It's a concentrated full spectrum hemp extract at this stage that looks like a gold-colored coconut fat and is now more than 50 percent fat and 25 percent CBD by volume. It's very powerful at this stage.

At this higher concentration, the mechanisms of action are through not only the endocannabinoid system, but much greater 5HT1a, TRPV, TRPA, TRPM, GABA, and PPAR receptor activation. This results in even more broad spectrum neurogenic support which may treat chronic pain, migraines, irritable bowel, fibromyalgia, cancer, addiction, treatment resistant conditions and is also beneficial in psychological health and wellness.

Consumers and practitioners have reported promising results with dosages of 3 to 60 mg daily of gold concentrated CBD oil extract. Dosages of 300 mg or greater of this CBD oil extract have been suggested for very serious and chronic conditions. As always, it is key to titrate the dose slowly to maximize efficacy while minimizing undesirable side effects such as drowsiness.

For best results, especially with difficult cases, always remember to titrate the dosage. This means you should increase slowly starting with gold CBD oil drops before soft-gels or concentrates to maximize response, while minimizing secondary effects like somnolence. Try integrating gold with raw hemp CBD oil extracts for the widest possible range of phytonutrients and phytocannabonoids. This combination is targeted for the most challenging treatment resistant situations.

Finally, formal safety studies of CBD oil extracts are lacking. One brand is purporting to have conducted formal toxicological safety data to support a Generally Recognized as Safe (GRAS) self-conclusion for 15 mg of CBD per day from a full spectrum Gold CBD hemp oil extract. FDA acknowledges the GRAS-self-conclusion process, if done properly and if successful may offer some more regulatory clarity and distinction between hemp and Marijuana products. However, as of the publishing of this guide no formal safety data on CBD has been reviewed and published in a journal since 1981.

To date, no hemp product has ever achieved anything close to GRAS status. To do so would be another monumental step in the acceptance of hemp extracts. The FDA would be in uncharted territory, as would the entire United States of America. All the evidence would point to hemp extract's safety and efficacy while none of the evidence would support prohibition or restriction of use. CBD could become both the wonder drug and nutritional ingredient of the twenty first century.

Some companies are marketing that botanical equivalents to hemp CBD can also be obtained without the use of the cannabis or hemp plant. This is patently false and may be misleading. Compounds known as *cannabimimetics* and other compounds found in extracts of ginger root, paeonia root, clove and echinacea and many other botanical sources do have some impact of the endocannabinoid system, but they are not nearly the same as CBD or THC. These clever products tout phytocannabinoids + cannabimimetics beta-caryophyllene + plant terpenes plant alkamides, however close inspection of the supplements fact panel reveals that they do not contain any CBD.

There are a number of CBD brands on the market, and it can be difficult to know what to look for when choosing a product that's right for you. Knowing the differences between the several types of CBD oils, the amount of CBD they deliver, and their source is the first step in choosing a product. The next thing to look for is brand transparency and understanding their supply chain process. Reading the label is also crucial in determining which type of oil you have and how much CBD, if any, is present. Lastly, quality should be a non-negotiable when it comes to making the right selection.

HOW THE OILS ARE SOLD

There is a growing number of hemp extracts now available in natural food stores, pharmacies, and online. They are available in many forms for a variety of uses. Before shopping for any specific products, you should consider which form is right for you. This includes the following:

Capsules and Softgels

These products mainly come in two forms: a capsule containing CBD oil that is spray dried onto rice flour as a green powder that is easily formulated and put into powders or capsules. Known as CBD oil capsules, they were the original full spectrum hemp derived CBD capsules in the market. Unintentionally confusing and counter intuitive, the original hemp oil that was dried and powdered are still available and effective.

The state-of-the-art delivery is ultimately soft gels made with vegetable gelatin and extra virgin olive oil to increase bioavailability by 3 fold. Softgels are available in a wide range of sizes and strengths, which should be taken as directed. The ingredients of the capsule itself may vary greatly. If formulated properly, these products contain the most precise serving sizes, in comparison to any other product.

CBD Drops and Sprays

Drops and sprays are available for full spectrum raw hemp liquid extracts, full spectrum activated hemp CBD oil extracts, and gold formula hemp CBD oil drops. Look for delicious gold formula peppermint drops sweetened with monk fruit. They tend to have the lowest amount of CBD per serving and can come in many flavors. Labels on all drops and sprays should be scrutinized, as some tinctures may contain harmful ingredients. Because drops and sprays are easy to manufacture and can be made at home, the quality of the product may be compromised. To avoid this, it is imperative to read the supplement facts panel and ask for a Certificate of Analysis (COA). The solution is to be taken orally, and normally sublingually—under the tongue.

Balms

The least invasive of all CBD products, topical balms are widely available and are normally applied to the skin. They may also be blended with other herbs and oils. While some products may be marketed as "transdermal," meaning absorbed through the skin, the science behind this kind of rub has not yet been fine-tuned and is considered a drug delivery system by FDA. The commercially available raw and gold balms can only be absorbed on the surface of the skin, similar to most lotions. Balms made with raw hemp oil extracts are reported to help with dry, itchy and flaky skin, even eczema and psoriasis.

Concentrates

This form is the most pure and natural way to administer any CBD product. They are pure concentrates free of any other added carrier oil or ingredient. Look for products that list other ingredients as "none" on the supplement facts panel to make sure it's a pure hemp extract concentrate. As mentioned in the previous section, there are many forms of CBD oil. Always pay attention to which type of oil is desired and make sure the label reflects that oil, whether it be sourced from marijuana or from certified agricultural hemp.

Vaporizers

These can refer to two types of inhalers: concentrate vaporizers and e-liquid vaporizers. Concentrate vaporizers are specifically designed to vaporize pure CBD concentrates that contain no added ingredients. Some CBD concentrates come prefilled in cartridges that attach to a vaporizer pen. There are also some specifically designed for the oil to be put directly onto the device for vaporization as well.

E-liquid CBD is also available in cartridge form. However, these cartridges usually contain other ingredients, mainly propylene glycol (PEG) or vegetable glycerin (VG). A less common ingredient that may also be used is polyethylene terephthalate resin (PET). Most of the time, CBD products containing PEG or PET should be avoided unless they are being used to quit or reduce combustion cigarette smoking or smokeless tobacco addiction. Risk reward benefits must always be carefully measured. Purified CBD vape shows tremendous promise for harm reduction and helping people break the crippling addiction to nicotine.

In addition to the products listed above, there are a number of other forms CBD comes in that you may wish to know more about. See the following inset for details. While it's good to find a product that you are comfortable using, there are a number of important factors to consider when evaluating one product from another. The next section will provide you with some important things to keep in mind when making your selection.

HOW THE OILS ARE EXTRACTED

There are several ways to draw the oil out of the hemp plant. The three which are most popular are the carbon dioxide method, the ethanol-based method, and the cold pressing method (which is typically only used for hemp seed oil). When any of these extraction methods use hemp that has been grown to high standards, the results should be clean oil.

Cold Pressing

Cold pressing is used when extracting oil from hemp seeds Here, the seeds, either whole or ground down, are put into a press where the oil is pressed out of the seeds. The heat created by friction should not exceed 120° F. This extraction method should only be used to extract oil from hemp seeds and is not helpful in producing oil high in cannabinoids, including CBD. This method is not likely to filter out any chemical impurities that the hemp seeds may contain.

Carbon Dioxide (CO2) Method

This method is one of the most popular, safe, and environmentally friendly extraction methods. It is the current standard for food and herbal supplements in the industry, where it is used for a variety of products, ranging from essential oils to decaffeinated coffee.

The hemp seed is placed under pressure with the carbon dioxide (CO_2) in order to extract the oils from the plant. After this process is complete, the CO_2 and the extract are moved from the pressure vessel to another location. In subcritical extraction, the CO_2 is placed at lower temperatures, and after passing through the extraction vessel, it is moved to an evaporator, where the CO_2 can return to a gas form and be released back into the atmosphere to be recycled. When supercritical CO_2 is used, the CO_2 is placed at higher temperatures, then separated from the extract after it goes through the extraction vessel. The extract then settles at lower temperatures. Once the CO_2 has cooled, it can be re-compressed and recycled, or released back into the atmosphere. Ideally, look for CBD that is extracted using the Carbon Dioxide (CO_2) method.

There are two ways this can be done:

One way is to put the solvent and plant material into an auger conveyor and separate the plant material from the extract. Another way is to spray the solvent of choice on the hemp as it enters the separation equipment, such as a centrifugal separator or belt press. In both cases, the "latency period" (the time between the combination of the solvent and the material, and the separation of the two) is a timed process where the temperature must be monitored to stay at cooler temperatures. After which, the extract and the solvent are quickly separated from each other. This process is not particularly harmful, but if not done properly the resulting oil may have some residual solvents present.

Solvents are used to convert cannabis or hemp that may not be fresh enough or clean enough to be extracted with cold pressing or carbon dioxide CO_2. They offer the possibility to extract commercially salable cannabinoids, even if the plant material is starting to rot and decompose. Even when producing 100 percent pure and natural isolated cannabinoids, solvent extraction is required.

Solvent extraction, especially butane, can produce widely coveted medical marijuana extracts, known as butane hash oil. These products are only legally sold in marijuana dispensaries. If the solvent-based extraction method is utilized with the intention of making full spectrum agricultural CBD oil extracts, insist on seeing third party test results proving the absence of any residual solvents, such as pentane and butane.

Most often, solvent extraction is used to make pure CBD crystals known as isolates. Isolates are just that, isolated CBD devoid of

A World of CBD Products

Today, there is a wide variety of CBD products available. As a customer it is important to check the source of the CBD and the amount of CBD in the product, perform potency testing to make sure the label meets claims, and check that the other ingredients that are present.

- CBD Apple Cider Vinegar
- CBD Lozenges
- CBD Chocolate Bars
- CBD Teas and Drinks
- CBD Coconut Oil
- CBD Water Soluble
- CBD Gum
- Isolated CBD Crystalline
- CBD Gummy Candies
- Natural and Propolis Healing Salve

nearly all cofactors and natural plant buffers. Isolates are the exact opposite of full spectrum hemp oil CBD extracts. They are closer to drugs and are not traditionally considered the kind of natural extract one would find in a health food store.

Based on the intellectual property rights surrounding pure CBD in addition to definitions of what technically differentiates a drug from a natural extract, isolated CBD crystals may end up only being available behind a pharmacy counter.

The bigger question with isolated CBD crystals is, are they actually synthetic or are the crystals natural? Properly made natural isolated CBD crystals can and fetch upwards of 50,000 per kilo for 99 percent pure CBD isolate.

Nanotechnology Delivery. Hemp CBD oil extracts produced with cold pressing, carbon dioxide (CO_2) method and even solvent-based extraction methods, may undergo additional processing with the promise of increased absorption or bioavailability. They can be sold under the names CBD water, water soluble CBD, liposomal, nanoemulsified or nanotechnology. These delivery systems may increase bioavailability in laboratory cell models and even in limited human studies. However, is it proof that we need less of these forms of CBD to get identical results from higher milligram amounts?

Products that claim to be 5 times more bioavailable than natural CBD oil extracts, for example, infer that only 2mg of enhanced absorption water soluble CBD or liposomal CBD will deliver the exact same effect as 10 mg of CBD from hemp oil extract. These claims are not proven to be accurate and are currently premature.

Remember that these delivery systems reduce the size of the droplet with the intent of driving the CBD deeper into tissues and through the body. If the starting material used is contaminated, even with non-detectable levels of toxins, aflatoxins, mold, fungus, heavy metals, solvents or worse synthetic CBD or CBD like analogs, the unknowns may outweigh perceived advantage over hemp extracts.

Thus, it's important to note that bioavailability and enhanced absorption claims of cannabinoids exceed the scientific data and may be more marketing than science.

THE GOOD, THE BAD, AND THE UGLY

Because of the gray area in which hemp products exist in the marketplace, by making sure you find the right product, you can reap the maximum benefits from this magnificent plant. The following points are essential to know when considering what product to buy.

Origin of the Products

Many countries throughout the world now produce hemp. While growing hemp may be good for these countries' economies, the problem for consumers using a hemp product is the uncertainty of what other unhealthful substances the plant may contain. In many of these hemp-growing nations, the rules for the use of dangerous pesticides and herbicides in growing these crops are lax or not stringently enforced. So while the original intent for growing these crops may not be for human consumption, many of these plants may find their way to secondary marketplaces that are specifically aimed at the health and beauty market.

Likewise, many quality manufacturers are committed to using certified hemp cultivars that are also used in the production of food grade hemp products. These food grade varieties of hemp are cultivated as agricultural crops and will prove to be ideal source of CBD.

In addition, the hemp plant is considered a "bioaccumulator." What this means is that the plant has the ability to absorb heavy metals and other chemical wastes found in the soil it grows in. Again, where the hemp is grown for non-human consumption should not be a problem; however, you may be putting yourself at risk by not knowing the origin of the hemp in the product you may be using.

To avoid this problem, it is important to ask the manufacturer for documentation on their hemp sourcing. Again, while the original purpose for growing hemp in most other countries was for fiber, there are varieties that are grown in a manner that is more targeted for nutrition and medical use. Typically, any manufacturer committed to quality and safety will gladly share this data with its consumers upon request. Knowing these facts can be illuminating. However, the savvy and discerning consumer knows that growing location or even certification fails to ensure toxicological safety at the recommended daily intake.

Hemp, like all plants, reflects the condition of its environment. The cleaner the environment, the cleaner the plant, the cleaner the product is in a logical refrain. Considering most consumers take between 5 to 15 mg of CBD per day from hemp CBD oil extracts, knowing that the ingested extract is proven fit for daily human consumption is the definitive test of safety.

According to a recent safety review published in *Cannabis and Cannabinoid Research*, "several aspects of a toxicological evaluation of a compound such as genotoxicity studies and research evaluating CBD effect on hormones are still scarce. Especially, chronic studies on CBD's effect on, for example, genotoxicity and the immune system, are still missing." They are very safe and non-toxic in humans. However, satisfying FDA's requirement of toxicological studies to investigate the safety of oral consumption of a new product to support a GRAS (Generally Recognized as Safe Status) self-conclusion is a different process than gaining organic certification, third party testing, or even human clinical trials with CBD.

These formal toxicology studies are required by law to introduce a new "food" into the human food supply. Hemp is ancient and hemp products have proven to be safe, yet hemp extracts are concentrated from whatever plant was used. The variables for contamination and exposure are troubling considering how much CBD will be required to meet the overwhelming demand.

Products that differentiate themselves with concerted evidence-based safety assessments required to obtain GRAS, which must be conducted at a GLP, FDA, OECD, EU, EC compliant toxicology lab. The substance needs to be proven not to be mutagenic, clastogenic, or genotoxic.

An established formula is to apply a 100-fold safety factor to determine if the serving size on the product is proven to be GRAS for the indented results. Look for a company's rating on the internet or through the Better Business Bureau (see Resource Section on page 00). You can also contact the company directly to ask questions or for actual copies of a certified organic license. While this is not always an easy task, it will be worth the effort. Several hemp seed oil and foods manufacturers have attained certified organic status. Some hemp growers are claiming to be growing on organically certified land. However, none of the hemp CBD oil extracts themselves are truly "Certified Organic," even if grown in complete accordance with all organic farming standards.

You may see the word "natural" on the label as well. Unfortunately, there is no real criteria for the use of the word. While it may refer to the fact that none of the ingredients in the product have been produced synthetically, it does not indicate that the hemp plant used has been certified organic. Without a legal definition, the word "natural" may simply be a marketing ploy to get your attention.

Other Active Ingredients

As more and more CBD products are made available, different manufacturers will add various other ingredients to their products. For example, today you will find not only plain CBD oils, but you will also find CBD tinctures (drops and sprays), CBD chocolate and gummies, Gold CBD in extra-virgin olive oil—the list goes on. These products are not pure CBD oil products, but formulations that contain CBD oil, mixed in carrier oils or other ingredients.

The most important thing to look out for in these particular products is the quality of the other ingredients, and if the CBD claim on the product matches the content in the actual formula. Have any additives been added for color enhancement or to make the product last longer? What chemicals or natural ingredients have been mixed in to make the product smell better? Does the company offer test results for the potency of their products?

While the CBD oil may not pose a problem in and of itself, another ingredient may cause an allergic reaction or may be problematic when taken with a specific prescription drug. It is therefore very important to carefully look at the label to see what ingredients the product contains. If you have questions about any of the ingredients in a product, ask a pharmacist or healthcare professional for help to determine the safety of a product you are not sure about.

What is the Shelf Life of CBD Extracts?

As a rule of thumb, CBD extracts will normally last in an unopened airtight bottle from twelve to eighteen months from the time of its manufacture. Once opened, it can last for another twelve months as long as it is stored in a dark bottle, kept in a cool area, and away from light. While it is most common to place opened bottles in the refrigerator, for some CBD products this is not recommended. As always, read the labels or contact the company if you are unsure of how to store your product.

Like any essential fatty oil, over a long period of time CBD oil will degrade, diminishing its therapeutic properties. It will also turn rancid when exposed to oxygen, light, and heat. Should the oil become oxidized, it would usually change to a darker color and give off an acrid odor, as though something was burning. It's important to throw out any oils that you believe have expired. The simplest way to avoid the possibility of the oil becoming rancid is to purchase one to three months' worth of oils at a time.

POTENCY

All CBD extract potency differs from one product to another. The level of potency is subject to several manufacturing factors:

1. The specific part or parts of the hemp plant used.

2. The extraction process used to draw out the oil.

3. The way the extracted oil may be concentrated.

4. The amount of other ingredients added to the extracted oil.

5. The ability for the manufacturer to standardize their oil production.

As mentioned earlier, any company that is properly manufacturing CBD products will have potency results from an independent testing lab and may also have results from their own laboratory analysis. Products such as sprays and drops (tinctures) will typically have lower concentrations of CBD per serving, because the oil is mixed in with other ingredients.

Some labels may claim to contain 1000 mg CBD in an entire bottle of product, but still only deliver as little as 1 mg per serving.

Softgels and capsules are also mixed with other ingredients but can contain up to 30 mg per softgel/capsule, and even more if made with isolated CBD crystals. Concentrated natural form, without any other ingredients, will typically have the highest milligram amount per serving.

If the milligram amount of CBD is not printed on the label it may confuse the consumer interested in how much CBD is in the bottle. Unfortunately, this is a regulatory tactic taken by uneducated or unscrupulous marketers of CBD products. With the hope of avoiding DEA, FDA, or DOJ enforcement, most sellers of hemp extracts today have elected to remove all references to cannabidiol CBD and the more potent peripheral anti-inflammatory cannabidiolic acid CBDA found in raw hemp oil extracts. Even sellers who do make ultra-high-quality food grade hemp extracts that are safe and effective may elect to eliminate any mention of CBD on the label until the Food and Drug Administration has an official position.

Just because the brand decides not to call out the cannabidiol (CBD) in the supplement facts panel does not mean that it's an inferior hemp extract. The only way to ensure the potency of the product as stated on the label is to acquire test results. These test results should ideally be from the manufacturer's in-house laboratory, along with corroborating third party testing for purity and potency from an accredited and respected independent laboratory.

The most valid and cutting critique of the burgeoning hemp extract industry are failed label claims. The majority of available CBD products today do not deliver the amount of CBD that is advertised. The FDA has the ability to liquidate a seller in the market who claims 15 mg per serving when it only contains 5 mg.

The analytical testing issue is further complicated once again because of the regulatory ambiguity of the cannabis hemp plant itself. This ambiguity is preventing the acceptance of cannabinoid testing standards, resulting in widely noted variation in cannabinoid content, even among accredited and respected laboratories. Groups like Consumer Lab have announced mass testing of CBD products and from existing data sets from laboratories that routinely test hundreds of brands. They have been tracking an 80 percent failure rate, meaning only 20 percent of the products tested actually contained what the consumer thought they were buying and more importantly getting for their health. In the end, no matter what it is, you only need to answer one simple question? Is CBD working for you?

IS CBD WORKING?

If you are taking CBD to treat a particular health problem, it is important to consult a healthcare professional. The bottom line is that you want the product to work, and that cannot always be determined without professional guidance. As you will see in the next section, there are many serious disorders that CBD has been shown to reduce in severity and even alleviate. There have been numerous medical studies published that have shown the effectiveness of CBD on many health issues.

However, it is important to point out that while CBD has proven to be effective in many cases, it may not work for everyone in the same way. First, our bodies are all different—from our unique DNA to the biochemistry that is us. This can make a big difference in outcome. Secondly, differing results can also stem from the specific product you are using to the amount you are taking. Therefore, before taking any CBD products to treat a health problem, it is important to consult a healthcare professional.

Once you are using CBD for any given problem, however, the fact is, you would also be the best judge to see if it is working. Over time, if it seems not to be helping, make sure that the oil you are using is the right oil. Consider changing the product to another brand. If you do not see or feel any positive changes over time, feel free to discontinue its use. Do not be afraid to look for other options that may provide potential relief.

A Buyer's Guide to CBD

The Many Benefits
of Cannabinoids and Terpenes

There are two important groups of compounds found in cannabis plants that researchers have found beneficial to our well-being. They are cannabinoids and terpenes.

Cannabinoids are natural compounds that are found in cannabis plants. The best known of these cannabinoids are THC and CBD. Now researchers have discovered over one hundred other cannabinoids, many of which also provide health benefits. Here are the top six cannabinoids along with what benefits they may provide.

Cannabidiol (CBD)

* Anti-diabetic
* Anti-epileptic
* Non-psychoactive

* Reduces nausea
* Reduces anxiety

Cannabichromene (CBC)

* Anti-inflammatory
* Anti-microbial
* Vasoconstriction
* Analgesic (Pain reliever)

* Antiprolferative (Used or tending to inhibit tumor cell growth)
* Non psychoactive

Cannabiovarin (CBD-V)

* Anti-emetic
* Anti-epileptic

* Bone stimulant
* Non psychoactive

Cannabinol (CBN)

* Anti-insomnia
* Anti-spasmodic

* Mildly psychoactive

Cannabigenol (CBG)

- Anti-bacterial
- Antiproliferative
- Bone stimulant
- Non psychoactive
- Neuroprotective and Neuromodulation which can reduce the severity of neurological disorders such as Parkinsons and Huntington diseases.

Cannabigerol A (CBGA)

Referred to as "Granddaddy of cannabinoids," scientists have known about CBG for over fifty years. Israeli researchers were the first to isolate the cannabinoid and thirty years later, Japanese scientists were the first to reveal that CBGA was its precursor.

- Acidic form of CBG, a precursor molecule to most cannabinoids. It is found in raw cannabis.
- When dried it converts to CBG.
- Helps in cardiovascular disease complications
- Helps in metabolic disorders
- In a recent computer stimulation study, CBGA was shown to help regulate metabolism.
- Can help treat colon cancer.

Terpenes are aromatic compounds. These terpene oils provide the pungent and fragrant odors of the plant. They also protect the plant from animal grazing and infectious germs. While they are found in many plants, they are highly concentrated in cannabis plants. There are over 120 terpenes in cannabis. While research is new, many terpenes have been found to provide a number of health benefits similar to cannabinoids. The scents some terpenes give off can also promote relaxation and stress-relief. Here are six terpenes along with what benefits they may provide.

Limonene

Gives the rinds of lemons and oranges their citrus smell.

- Anti-inflammatory
- Antioxidant
- Antiviral
- Anti-diabetic
- Anti-cancer

Pinene

Pine Tree scent

- Allows more air in the lungs
- Anti-inflammatory
- Bronchodilator

Linolool

Important compound in Aromatherapy

- Anti-anxiety
- Anti-cancer
- Anti-depressant
- Anti-inflammatory
- Anti-microbial
- Calming effect (Lavender)
- Neuro protective

Mycene

- Anti-inflammatory
- Antioxidant
- Studies used high doses up to 200 mg kg of weight.

Beta-caryophylene

- Anti-inflammatory

Humulene

- May prevent allergic reactions and asthma.

CONCLUSION

"Let the buyer beware" is an important phrase to keep in mind when looking for most any products. As someone who may be trying to overcome a health issue, this phrase is doubly important. Today, there are many unsubstantiated claims floating around the internet—many designed to sell products. Unfortunately, hype is no substitute for facts. As a customer looking for the best product, your job is to become a smart consumer. By taking the time to learn the facts, you will be in a better position to ask the right questions and make informed decisions. Hopefully this guide will help you on your journey to a healthier you.

An Alphabetical Guide to Using CBD

C BD is available in a number of concentrations and forms, such as liquid oil; concentrate balms; vapor from vaporizers; easy to take and convenient vegetarian softgels capsules, sublingual tinctures, drops or sprays with extra virgin olive oil; even edibles in the form of candy. Topical CBD balms may also be effective for acne. Treatment resistant skin conditions may require much higher concentrations and in this application, isolated CBD crystals may prove to be ideal.

ADDICTION, OPIATE

Opiate addiction is a serious problem in the US today. Opiates include a vast assortment of drugs, ranging from legal drugs such as fentanyl, codeine, and morphine, to illegal drugs such as heroin and opium. Over a period of time people become physically reliant on these drugs. This addiction can occur if the drugs are prescribed by a doctor or if they are being used illegally.

Symptoms

An indication of an opiate addiction is when an individual continues using even when they are aware that there are negative consequences. Some physical signs of this addiction are characterized by:

- Constipation
- Constricted pupils
- Drowsiness/marked sedation
- Elation

- Euphoria
- Loss of consciousness
- Mood swings
- Noticeable confusion

Triggers

What may trigger drug use and/or abuse for one individual may be different for someone else. However, the following are triggers that are common to most people:

- Anxiety
- Chronic illness
- Chronic pain
- Depression

- Frustration
- Rejection
- Stress

Conventional Treatment/Side Effects

There are now drugs available to treat opiate addictions. They are categorized as *agonists* and *partial agonists*, which act like opiates but are safer and less addictive, and *antagonists*, which block the addictive effects of opiates. But they are not without side effects. Agonists such as methadone, hydrocodone bitartrate, and oxycodone hydrochloride may have similar side effects as heroin and may trigger depressed breathing. Buprenorphine, a partial agonist, may cause nausea and constipation. Naltrexone, an antagonist, may block pain relief if you are using an opiate medication for pain.

Benefits of CBD

Research has shown that CBD has "a very low abuse potential and inhibits drug-seeking behavior." In an animal study, researchers found that the effects of CBD lasted as long as two weeks after it was administered, while methadone needed to be administered daily to be effective. The potential of CBD's effect on decreasing the opiate addiction "by lowering its overall effect on the central nervous system" was also cited in the study.

In 2017, there were ninety-one deaths from opiate overdose a day in the US. CBD is a plant, not a man-made drug. It is not addictive and has minimal side effects at recommended doses. As stated in a 2015 report by the Partnership for Drug-Free Kids, "there are hundreds of people in Massachusetts being treated with medical pot in order to control their addiction to opioids. There have been so many opiate-linked deaths in the state that doctors are getting patients on to non-addictive cannabis [CBD] as much as they can to stop more fatalities from occurring."

Dr. Dustin Sulak, the founder and director of Integr8 Health stated: "In addition to keeping people in treatment, replacing and reducing the opioids, improving the pain relief that opioids provide, and preventing opioid dose escalation and tolerance, cannabis can also treat the symptoms of opioid withdrawal: nausea, vomiting, diarrhea, abdominal cramping, muscle spasms, anxiety, agitation, restlessness, insomnia, and also minor symptoms like runny nose and sweating."

How to Use

Recommended dosage is 15 to 50 mg multiple times daily. CBDA, CBD, and other cannabinoids represent a new group of natural anti-addiction agents. CBD is currently being developed as a drug to treat smokeless tobacco addiction. The initial findings are remarkable and the future for these natural plant-based signaling molecules or extracts to address multiple forms of addiction should be considered.

ADHD

See **ATTENTION DEFICIT HYPERACTIVITY DISORDER.**

AGE-RELATED MACULAR DEGENERATION

Age-related macular degeneration (AMD) generally impacts older adults, over the age of 60. It is a medical disease affecting the eye, generating a loss of vision in the macula (the center of the visual field) because of damage that has occurred to the retina. There are two forms of AMD:

Dry AMD. This form develops from atrophy to the retinal pigment epithelial layer below the retina.

Wet AMD. This form occurs due to abnormal blood vessel growth causing damaging and rapid vision loss if not treated.

Symptoms

You may not experience any symptoms in the early stages of AMD; however, the first sign of the condition may be characterized by a gradual or sudden change in the quality of your vision. Other symptoms may include:

- Changes in perception of color, in rare cases
- Dark, blurry areas
- Loss of central vision
- Whiteout in the center of your vision

Conventional Treatment/Side Effects

Although there is no cure for this disease, drugs like Lucentis and Avastin have been used to slow or prevent increased loss of vision. Injections in the eye, such as Macugen and Eylea, may also be pre-scribed to slow down the loss of vision. Even though these treatments have been FDA-approved for treating AMD, there may be possible serious side effects associated with their use, such as:

- Bleeding (bloodshot eye) or discharge from the eye
- Eye infections
- Eye pain, redness

- Flashes of light or floaters
- Retinal detachment
- Sensitivity to light
- Swelling around the eyes
- Swelling of the cornea
- Vision problems

In addition to the use of drugs as a treatment, laser surgery is another option.

Benefits of CBD

Correlations have been cited between the healing power of CBD and workings of age-related macular degeneration. In a Finnish study published in the journal *Pharmacology & Therapeutics* in 2002, the researchers observed that the eye has cannabinoid receptors. The study concluded that "smoking cannabis directly was found to lower intraocular pressure in glaucoma patients."

CB1 receptors in the endocannabinoid system affect the area of the eye that is responsible for eye pressure. CB2 receptors affect the retina and the cornea. It is probable that these molecules can positively affect these particular tissues, and conceivably, the progression of AMD. More research is needed to show details of these receptors and how the tissues react to these molecules.

Cannabinoids have been shown to help AMD symptoms. Research has cited that cannabinoids:

- Are anti-inflammatory for the retina area
- Are neuro-protective
- Are anti-angiogenesis
- Have anti-aging properties
- Inhibit VEGF growth (vascular endothelial growth factor), the growth of new blood vessels
- Lowers blood pressure
- Protects retina cells
- Reduce ocular pressure

How to Use

Recommended dosage is 3 to 30 mg daily. THC may also be needed in some cases, provided the patient can tolerate THC. If not, a larger dose of CBD may be effective, up to 120 mg per day. Omega 3 ALA in addition to marine omega 3 EPA and DHA may enhance benefits.

If you are trying an enhanced delivery system form of CBD and not achieving the desired results, then take the same milligram serving from a hemp extract that lists the milligram amount of CBD on the label. Analytical purity and potency results that are validated by non-negotiable third party independent results corroborate precisely how much CBD per serving you are really getting.

ALZHEIMER'S DISEASE

Alzheimer's disease is a progressive brain disorder that gradually brings about the destruction of large numbers of nerve cells in the brain. It slowly impairs memory and thinking skills and eventually leads to an inability to carry out simple tasks. Medical experts suggest that over 5 million Americans may have been diagnosed with Alzheimer's disease in the US. At the present time it is ranked as the sixth leading cause of death.

Symptoms

In the beginning, the only symptom that may be noticeable is forgetfulness, confusion, or difficulty organizing your thoughts. However, as the disease progresses the changes in the brain may lead to:

- Behavior changes
- Confusion with time
- Changes in mood
- Difficulty forming judgments and making decisions
- Difficulty planning

- Difficulty carrying out and completing familiar tasks
- Difficulty thinking and reasoning
- Disruptive memory loss
- Personality changes
- Problems speaking
- Withdrawal from social interest

Triggers

Scientists still don't have a completely clear understanding of what causes Alzheimer's disease in most people, however they believe that genetics, lifestyle, and environmental factors come into play. Over time these elements may affect the brain. Evidence suggests many theories that may put you at risk for developing Alzheimer's, including the following factors:

- Age
- Diabetes, type 2
- Diet
- Drugs
- Exposure to toxic substances
- Genetics
- Head injury
- High blood pressure
- High cholesterol level
- Lack of exercise
- Obesity
- Sleep deprivation
- Smoking

Conventional Treatment/Side Effects

Currently, the two medications most commonly prescribed as a treatment for Alzheimer's are cholinesterase inhibitors and memantine. The effectiveness of these drugs differ from person to person.

Cholinesterase inhibitors and memantine drugs may slow down the progression of the disease, but not without side effects. The cholinesterase inhibitors may cause nausea, vomiting, appetite loss, or frequent bowel movements; in particular, the drug donepezil has been associated with seizures. Memantine drugs may result in headaches, constipation, confusion, and dizziness.

Scientists are searching to find new treatments because the current treatments mask the symptoms, but do not treat the underlying disease. In 2006, *The New York Times* cited a study done by *The New England Journal of Medicine* which indicated that "drugs most commonly used to soothe agitation and aggression in people with Alzheimer's disease are no more effective than placebos for most patients, and put them at risk of serious side effects, including confusion, sleepiness, and Parkinson's disease-like symptoms, researchers are reporting today." There is no cure, prevention, or treatment to slow the advancement of Alzheimer's.

Benefits of CBD

The starting point for change to evolve in the medical treatment of Alzheimer's is the acknowledgment that today's treatments are not safe or effective, and although they may reduce symptoms, the conventional drug cannot reverse or slow down the progression of the disease. CBD has been shown to reverse cognitive deficits of Alzheimer's transgenic mice. A study cited in a 2014 issue of the *Journal of Alzheimer's Disease* was the earliest to give evidence of CBD's ability to avert the occurrence of a social recognition deficit in AD transgenic mice. According to the study, "control and Alzheimer's transgenic mice were treated orally from 2.5 months of age with CBD (20 mg/kg) for 8 months. Mice were then assessed in the social preference test, elevated plus maze, and fear conditioning paradigms, before cortical and hippocampal tissues were analyzed for amyloid load, oxidative damage, cholesterol, phytosterols, and inflammation. [The researchers] found that AβPP x PS1 mice developed a social recognition deficit, which was prevented by CBD treatment." The data gives [them] initial evidence that CBD may be viable as a preventative treatment for Alzheimer's symptoms such as social withdrawal and facial recognition.

Research has shown that CBD aides in neurogenesis, the generation of new neurons in the hippocampus area of the brain. It is in this part of the brain where memory is formed, organized, and stored. This is crucial since neurons play an important role in the transmission of messages within the brain as well as throughout the nervous system. CBD can help to prevent the formation of Alzheimer's plaques in the brain.

Dr. David Schubert, a professor at the Salk Institute, studied the effects of cannabinoids on Alzheimer's treatment. His findings show that CBD may reduce the amount of beta-amyloid, a protein fragment commonly thought to cause the neurodegenerative disease in the brain. He stated: "Although other studies have offered evidence that cannabinoids might be neuroprotective against the symptoms of Alzheimer's, we believe our study is the first to demonstrate that cannabinoids affect both inflammation and amyloid beta accumulation in nerve cells."

How to Use

Recommended dosage is 330 mg. Some reports suggest marijuana has been shown to slow and even reverse Alzheimer's in rats. THC may be effective, if tolerated. Check with healthcare provider before using cannabis or THC products. Taking small amounts of CBD when feelings of stress and anxiety are high have also been reported.

AMD

See **AGE-RELATED MACULAR DEGENERATION.**

ANXIETY DISORDERS

The occasional occurrence of anxiety is a normal part of life. However, when it occurs more frequently and causes such distress that it restricts your ability to function and gets in the way of leading a normal life, anxiety can become disabling and a serious mental disorder. Anxiety can present itself in various ways, such as panic attacks, phobias, and social fears. It has been established that anxiety and related disorders affect about 40 million adults aged eighteen and older.

Symptoms

Anxiety disorders are characterized by symptoms that appear suddenly and become so chronic that they disrupt our daily lives. These symptoms include:

- Chest pain
- Feeling of choking
- Heart palpitations
- Inability to relax
- Muscle tension
- Poor concentration
- Sweating
- Upset stomach

Triggers

A number of factors may trigger anxiety. The causes or risk factors for generalized anxiety disorders (GAD) may include:

- Caffeine
- Family history of anxiety
- Family illnesses
- Fears
- Illnesses
- Stressful situations, severe or long-lasting

Conventional Treatment/Side Effects

Most physicians prescribe selective serotonin reuptake inhibitors (SSRIs) or serotonin norepinephrine reuptake inhibitors (SNRIs) as treatment for anxiety disorders. Some feel that these medications should be supplemented with cognitive-behavioral therapy (CBT) to be most effective. Prescription anxiety mediations such as SSRIs may result in weight gain, insomnia, and sexual dysfunction.

Antidepressants have proven to increase the risk of suicide in adolescents up to twenty-four years of age.

Benefits of CBD

Evidence gathered from animal studies and human experimental, clinical, and epidemiological studies point to elements in CBD that may be favorable in treating various anxiety-related conditions, including:

- Depression
- Obsessive Compulsive Disorder
- Panic disorders
- Post-Traumatic Stress
- Social fears (phobia)

Like SSRIs, CBD may also target the serotonin system by helping the brain cells transmit more serotonin signals, which help to alleviate anxiety and heighten mood.

In an animal study, Spanish researchers studied the effects of 3 to 45 mg of CBD daily. Omega 3 ALA in addition to marine omega 3 EPA and DHA may enhance benefits.

APPETITE LOSS

A decreased or loss of appetite occurs when you have a reduced desire to eat and dulled taste buds. While a healthy appetite is characteristic of positive health, loss of appetite may be a sign of a number of problems.

Symptoms

The primary symptoms associated with a loss of appetite are malnutrition and unintentional weight loss. Fatigue and loss of appetite combined leads to dizziness, fainting, blurry vision, lethargy, and a racing heartbeat. If left untreated, these conditions may become serious.

Triggers

A variety of conditions or diseases may lead to a loss of appetite. It can be triggered by physical illness or mental illness. Feelings of grief, depression, and anxiety can also stifle the appetite. Some of the conditions may be serious, such as certain cancers, chronic liver disease, kidney failure, thyroid disorders, infection, or dementia. Appetite loss is also a potential side effect of a number of medications, including antidepressants and antibiotics.

Conventional Treatment/Side Effects

Most commonly prescribed drugs for appetite loss include anti-emetics, which are typically recommended for nausea and vomiting, and antihistamines. Although these medications enhance the appetite, they generally cause a wide range of negative side effects.

Benefits of CBD

Although research into the benefits of CBD and appetite loss is still in the early stages, one of the significant benefits researchers have found is the use of CBD as a digestive aid. Studies suggest that cannabinoid receptors play a crucial role in controlling eating behavior. When CBD binds to C1 receptors, it stimulates the appetite while easing nausea and vomiting. This has been especially helpful for treating patients undergoing chemotherapy, as well as other serious diseases. Cannabinoids may also assist in dealing with emotional disorders, which affects one's interest in food.

How to Use

According to the Mayo Clinic, the suggested dosage to increase appetite in cancer patients is 2.5 milligrams of THC by mouth with or without 1 mg of CBD for six weeks. As the dosage of CBD differs for each person, it is best to start small and gradually increase until you experience the desired result.

ARTHRITIS

Arthritis is an inflammatory condition that can affect one or multiple joints. It occurs when the immune system begins to attack healthy joints. Although there are many different types of arthritis, the three most common are osteoarthritis, rheumatoid arthritis, and psoriatic arthritis. Osteoarthritis occurs most often and is characterized by the wear and tear of overused joints; rheumatoid arthritis materializes when the immune system strikes parts of the body causing inflammation and damage to the joints; and psoriatic arthritis is a condition defined by an inflammation of the skin and joints.

Symptoms

Commonly, the symptoms and signs are associated with the joints. Depending on the kind of arthritis you have, you may experience:

- Decreased range of motion
- Muscle and joint pain
- Fatigue
- Stiffness
- Joint redness and warmth
- Swelling

Most types of arthritis are triggered by a combination of varied factors.

Triggers

Again, the cause of arthritis pain depends on the type or form of arthritis you have. There is no single cause for the hundreds of kinds of arthritis. Common factors that may be potential causes may include:

- Abdominal pain
- Immune system dysfunction
- Fatigue
- Infection Injury
- Genetics
- Stress

Conventional Treatment/Side Effects

Nonsteroidal anti-inflammatory drugs (NSAIDs) may aid in alleviating pain and inflammation in the various kinds of arthritis, but they are associated with a number of side effects, including stomach bleeding. They also pose the risk of cardiovascular problems, such as heart attack and stroke.

Acetaminophen, brand name Tylenol, has anti-pyretic (anti-fever) properties and relieves arthritis pain as well. However, it can trigger liver and kidney problems. Steroids may also decrease inflammation, but they increase the risk of infection and cataracts and may result in weakened bones. Disease-modifying anti-rheumatic drugs (DMARDs) decelerate—but do not reverse—joint damage, which can bring about side effects, such as increased risk of serious infection.

Benefits of CBD

In a rodent study, researchers discovered that CBD was effective in lessening inflammation and pain associated with arthritis, leading them to the conclusion that CBD has potential in treating chronic pain. In this study, the researchers observed both inflammatory and neuropathic pain.

Doctors have cited that cannabinoid oil plays a role in the treatment of all types of arthritis. In a study conducted in 2006, patients suffering from rheumatoid arthritis who used cannabinoid oil for a period of 5 weeks experienced less pain and reduced inflammation.

A 2013 study published in *Rheumatology* found that both CBD and THC engage with CB2 receptors and that "CBD increases the amount of endocannabiniods in the body. By directly engaging with the endocannabinoid system, cannabis taps into the body's own system of self-repair. The herb calms inflammation and reigns in the immune system, giving your nerves and tissue some time to recover."

Aging arthritis patients find bone health crucial to their well-being. CBD has been proven to stimulate bone regeneration and to provide protection to other bones in the skeletal system. The *Journal of Bone Health* cited a study carried out by Dr. Yankel Gabet that showed that "CBD alone promotes 'markedly advanced' healing in broken bones by enhancing and speeding up the maturation of the collagenous matrix in the bone, a microstructure which provides the basis for mineralization of new bone tissue. With CBD therapy, according to Dr. Gabet's study, the broken bones will not only heal faster, but be harder to break than a bone left untreated with CBD."

Treating arthritis with CBD is a favorable step in the healing and treatment of rheumatoid arthritis and osteoarthritis. Since cannabinoids not only restores bone damage, but also manage pain and reduces tension. It is a desirable choice for suffering arthritics who want to find an alternative plan of treatment.

How to Use

According to the Mayo Clinic, the dosage recommended to treat chronic pain is 3 to 30 mg of CBD by mouth for an average of twenty-five days. Raw CBDA rich hemp extracts may also be effective. It is recommended to take anywhere from one to six servings (5 mg capsules or soft-gels) of CBDA daily. Omega 3 ALA in addition to marine omega 3 EPA and DHA may enhance benefits.

ATTENTION DEFICIT HYPERACTIVITY DISORDER

Attention deficit hyperactivity disorder (ADHD) is a common condition generally characterized by an inability to stay focused, pay attention, and control behavior. It is typically diagnosed in childhood but sometimes persists through adolescence and adulthood. ADHD affects about 11 percent of school-aged children and 2 to 5 percent of adults in the US today.

It is important to note that in 1994, attention deficit disorder (ADD) was changed to "attention-deficit hyperactivity disorder," regardless of whether the individual showed symptoms of hyperactivity or not. The three types of ADHD are now identified as "predominately hyperactive-impulsive," "predominately inattentive," and "combined." A great many professionals and laypeople alike still use both terms, ADD and ADHD, interchangeably.

Symptoms

ADHD manifests itself differently in everyone. Other signs of the disorder may include:

- Excessive talking
- Hyperactivity
- Fidgeting
- Impulsivity
- Forgetfulness
- Making careless mistakes
- Disorganization

Triggers

Although there is no specific cause for these disorders, research has indicated that certain factors, such as genetics, environment, and brain injury, may play a role. In the majority of cases, children diagnosed with ADHD have a relative that has also been diagnosed with the condition. Exposure to toxic levels of lead has also been shown to contribute to ADHD.

Research has also suggested that there is a connection between nutrition and diet and ADHD symptoms. It is believed that food additives and sugar as well as a lack of omega-3 fatty acids may contribute to these symptoms.

Conventional Treatment/Side Effects

Generally, ADHD is treated with short-acting and long-acting stimulants, nonstimulants, and antidepressants. Stimulants, such as Ritalin, Adderall, and Dexedrine are the most common type of medication prescribed.

In the late 1990s, researchers discovered that methylphenidate, the active ingredient in Ritalin, treats ADHD symptoms by increasing dopamine levels in the brain. However, it was also discovered that Ritalin had a significant potential to cause permanent brain damage and psychiatric problems. Even non-stimulant ADHD drugs have serious psychiatric problems.

Although these stimulants may be effective in controlling and reducing the symptoms, as mentioned above, there are some harmful side effects. Signs that may indicate problems are:

- Decreased appetite
- Delayed growth
- Headaches
- Irritability
- Moodiness
- Sleep problems
- Stomach aches

Benefits of CBD

Medical studies have demonstrated CBD's ability to reduce cortisol levels in the brain, which naturally causes an increase in dopamine levels. The results in treating ADHD with cannabis are often very significant.

Research cites grades going from C's and D's to A's and B's. In almost all cases ADHD patients who were treated with cannabis gave an account of how it helped them pay attention, focus their attention, and stay on task. Dr. Bearman, a "figurehead of cannabis research," examined the relationship between the cannabinoid system and ADHD. His studies influenced the findings of the prospective therapeutic value of cannabinoids, which improve the brain's dopamine management systems.

How to Use

For a number of reasons, it is important to start slow and go slow. Starting with small amounts allows you more control in finding the optimum dose.

Administer CBD 2 hours apart from pharmaceuticals to help avert adverse medication interactions. To aid in its absorption, it should be taken with a high fat snack. Oils can be taken by syringe, in capsules, and through G-tubes. Less is often more with these situations and large amounts of CBD can cause anxiety in some cases. Look for a 100-mg spray product or drop that can deliver CBD per milligram. Some doctors have reported benefit with only a few sprays or 1 to 3 mg of CBD.

BLOOD CLOTS

Blood clots are clumps of blood that form as a result of an injury or cut, most commonly in the limbs. They can also form inside veins and arteries. If the clots break off, they may become embedded in the heart, lungs, or brain. Clots forming inside your arteries may prevent oxygen from getting to your heart, lungs, or brain, resulting in life-threatening conditions.

Symptoms

Blood clots give differing symptoms depending on where in the body they appear. Many times, blood clots will exist without any symptoms:

Leg or Arm

- Change in color
- Pain
- Swelling
- Tenderness
- Warm sensation

Heart

- Lightheadedness
- Severe pain in chest and/or arm
- Shortness of breath
- Sweating

Lungs

- Chest pain
- Coughing up blood
- Feeling dizzy
- Heart palpitations
- Problems breathing
- Shortness of breath
- Sweating

Brain

- Difficulty seeing
- Difficulty speaking
- Sudden, severe headache

Abdomen

- Bloody stools
- Diarrhea
- Nausea
- Severe pain and swelling
- Vomiting

Triggers

Decrease in blood flow caused by clots may result in significant health problems. There are a number of risk factors and conditions that result from the formation of blood clots, such as:

- Cancer and cancer treatments
- Dehydration
- Family history
- Immobility, prolonged
- Irregular heartbeat
- Medications
- Obesity
- Oral contraception
- Pregnancy
- Smoking

- Stroke
- Surgery

- Varicose veins

Conventional Treatment/Side Effects

Most commonly, blot clots are treated with anticoagulants or blood thinners. They prevent the clots from progressing and slow down the stretch of time it takes for blood to clot. The blood thinner most frequently prescribed is UF Heparin.

Although anticoagulants prevent new clots from forming and existing clots from growing, they may result in complications, such as internal bleeding, bruising, skin irritation at the sight of injection, bluish colored skin, and itching of the feet. If used over a long period of time, anticoagulants may cause osteoporosis.

Benefits of CBD

Hemp oil is a natural blood thinner due to its omega-3 properties, helping to shorten and prevent blood clots. According to *Medical Marijuana Research*, "hemp could increase the anticoagulant effect of blood thinners by inhibiting its metabolism. It directly affects the anticoagulant properties of platelets in the blood. Therefore it naturally acts as a blood thinner and should rather be a replacement for blood thinning meds."

How to Use

If you are on blood thinners and would like to switch to CBD, it is advisable to do so under the supervision of a physician. It is also important to take note that extracts with 2:1 THC to CBD ratio have been reported to be effective. Recommended dosage is between 3 mg to 30 mg of CBD taken daily.

See also: **HEADACHES; HEART DISEASE.**

CANCER

There are over a hundred different types of cancer. Cancer occurs when the cells in a body region begin dividing and spreading into surrounding tissues. It can appear anywhere inside the body. Many cancers form solid masses of tissue called *tumors*. There are two types of tumors: benign and malignant. Cancerous tumors are malignant and can invade or spread to nearby tissue. Benign tumors do not spread or invade nearby tissue, but they can be fairly large and depending upon their location, they can be life-threatening.

Symptoms

At the early stages of the cancer there may not be any noticeable signs or symptoms; however, as the disease develops, symptoms or signs may appear depending upon the cancer type, the stage, and the location. Common symptoms may include:

- Change in bowel habits
- Change in urination
- Fatigue
- Fever
- Loss of appetite
- Nausea
- Pain

- Persistent cough
- Skin changes
- Unexplained anemia
- Unusual lumps or discharge
- Vomiting
- Unexpected weight loss or weight gain

Triggers

Most cancers are due to environmental factors, while about 5 to 10 percent are due to genetic factors. This abnormal cell growth may be caused by the following:

- Autoimmune diseases
- Chemicals (carcinogens)

- Chronic inflammation
- Diet

- Genetics
- Hormones
- Infection
- Physical inactivity
- Radiation
- Smoking

Conventional Treatment/Side Effects

There are a number of conventional treatments for cancer. The kind of treatment prescribed will depend on the type of cancer and how advanced it is. These treatments include:

- Chemotherapy
- Hormone therapy
- Immunotherapy
- Precision medicine
- Radiation therapy
- Stem cell transplant
- Surgery
- Targeted therapy

There are problems or side effects that appear when conventional cancer treatments affect healthy tissues or organs. Common side effects caused by cancer treatment may include:

- Anemia
- Appetite loss
- Bladder problems
- Bleeding (low platelets)
- Bruising easily
- Constipation
- Delirium
- Diarrhea
- Edema (water retention)
- Fatigue
- Hair Loss (Alopecia)
- Low white blood cells
- Lymphedema
- Mouth and throat problems
- Nerve problems (Peripheral Neuropathy)
- Pain
- Problem concentrating
- Sexual and fertility problems
- Skin and nail changes
- Urinary problems
- Vomiting

Benefits of CBD

Cannabinoids offer patients a healing alternative in the treatment of extremely invasive cancers. Over twenty major research studies show that cannabinoids have anti-cancer properties with the potential to stop the growth of several different types of cancers, including melanoma, brain cancer, and breast cancer. Cannabinoids may also offset chemical toxicity from drugs and environmental sources, helping to preserve normal cells. Researchers at the University of Milan found that cannabidiol inhibits the growth of glioma cells, a type of brain tumor, in a dose-dependent manner, selectively targeting and killing malignant cells. Certain CBD products have been approved in treating cancer pain in Canada and parts of Europe.

The medical establishment has also recognized the benefits of CBD for the side effects of chemotherapy. Studies have found that THC may also be advisable if the patient can tolerate it. Seek the guidance of a qualified healthcare provider with a proven track record and understanding of cannabinoids and cancer. Self-medication is ill advised and is not recommended.

How to Use

Try to obtain the highest quality of CBD possible. Find a broad-spectrum CBD oil in tinctures or gel capsules. Begin with a dosage of between 20 mg to 40 mg daily and then raise the dose in 10 mg increments until relief is felt.

CARDIOVASCULAR DISEASE

See **HEART DISEASE.**

CHEMOTHERAPY, SIDE EFFECTS

See **CANCER.**

COLITIS, ULCERATIVE

See **ULCERATIVE COLITIS.**

CROHN'S DISEASE

Crohn's disease is a chronic, recurring inflammatory bowel disease (IBD) that primarily affects the lining of the gastrointestinal (GI) tract. Since the disease involves the immune system you may experience joint pain, eye problems, a skin rash, or liver disease. Crohn's can be painful and debilitating. With treatment, however, Crohn's patients can keep the disease in check.

Symptoms

Crohn's may be characterized by the following symptoms and signs ranging from mild to severe:

- Abdominal pain
- Anal fissures
- Anemia
- Bloody stools
- Fever
- Malnutrition
- Nausea
- Obstruction in the bowel
- Weight loss

Triggers

The exact cause of Crohn's disease is unknown. Possible factors leading to the development of the disease have been connected to a combination of several elements, including problems with the immune system, genetics, and the environment.

Conventional Treatment/Side Effects

There is no cure for Crohn's disease. Medications are prescribed to control or prevent inflammation, and the choice of medication depends on the severity of the disease and whether complications exist.

Anti-inflammatory drugs are usually prescribed first, such as oral 5-aminosalicylates and corticosteroids (prednisone). Some side effects associated with anti-inflammatory drugs are upset stomach, nausea, vomiting, headache, dizziness, loss of appetite, and/or fatigue.

Immune system suppressors, such as Stelera, Tysabri, and Rheumatrex, also reduce inflammation. However, they should not be used long-term because of side effects, such as bloating, excessive facial hair, sleep disruption, and heightened risk of developing diabetes and osteoporosis.

When an infection is a consideration, antibiotics are prescribed, but there is no strong proof that they are effective for treating Crohn's disease. Common side effects experienced when taking an antibiotic include diarrhea, upset stomach, and nausea.

Benefits of CBD

Cannabinoids have been found to lessen inflammation in the bowel, eventually reducing pain, providing nausea relief, and reducing feelings of unpleasantness. Present-day discoveries indicate that cannabinoid treatments are a significant competitor in the therapy and remission of Crohn's disease.

In a 2005 pilot study, Tod Mikuriya, MD, and David Bearman, MD, questioned twelve Crohn's patients taking cannabis about their post-treatment symptoms. The patients reported a vast improvement in overall symptoms without adverse side effects.

How to Use

Recommended dosage is 3 to 30 mg daily. The reduction of stress and anxiety are critical for sufferers of inflammatory bowel disease.

DEPRESSION

We have all felt sad or down at one time or another, but sadness becomes problematic when it persists and negatively affects our life. Depression is one of the most common mental disorders. It is a mood disorder that affects almost all aspects of daily life. It may impact how you think, how you feel, and daily activities, such as sleeping, eating, and working.

Symptoms

According to the American Psychiatric Association, depression is characterized by "a deep feeling of sadness or a marked loss of interest or pleasure in activities." Common symptoms that usually are associated with depression may include:

- Change in appetite
- Chronic fatigue
- Excessive sleep or insomnia
- Feeling lethargic
- Feelings of hopelessness and worthlessness
- Inability to focus
- Lack of appetite or eating too much
- Loss of interest in sex
- Loss of interest in social activities and daily activities
- Moodiness
- Restlessness and irritability
- Thoughts of suicide
- Unexplained aches and pains
- Unexplained crying and anger outbursts

Triggers

Research has made clear that depression is a serious illness caused by changes in brain chemistry. Many factors can contribute to the onset of depression, including genetics, changes in hormone levels, certain medical conditions, stress, grief, difficult life circumstances, or substance abuse. The depression may be triggered by one or a combination of factors.

Conventional Treatment/Side Effects

Traditionally, treatment for depression includes forms of psycho-therapy and/or medications. There are a number of forms of psy-chotherapy that are used, such as cognitive-behavioral therapy (CBT), which works to replace negative thought patterns with more grounded and useful ones.

The most common medications prescribed are called selective serotonin re-uptake inhibitors (SSRIs). Prozac (fluoxetine), Paxil (paroxetine), Zoloft (sertraline) and Luvox (fluvoxamine) are the most popular brands. Although SSRI antidepressant medications seem to be safe, many people will experience side effects while taking them, such as nausea, diarrhea, agitation, insomnia, head-ache, or decreased sex drive. Long-term side effects of taking SSRI medications may include difficulties sleeping, sexual dysfunction, and weight gain.

Benefits of CBD

The endocannabinoid system in our brain helps to balance mood and influence our "reward-seeking behavior." It also helps main-tain balance in the body by reducing stress and regulating sleep and appetite. Depression can negatively impact the endocannabi-noid system, resulting in poor sleep and eating habits, as well as high levels of stress. Researchers at the University of Buffalo have found that using cannabidiol to restore endocannabinoid function may help to stabilize mood and treat depression. Cannabis use has been proven to ease stress, help insomnia, and regulate appetite.

Although anyone can use CBD to manage depression, it is advisable to consult your doctor or medical caregiver if you are pregnant or suffering from other diseases. If you are considering changing from traditional pharmaceuticals to CBD, it is also important to solicit advice from your physician or medical caregiver.

How to Use

Recommended dosage is 3 to 45 mg. Raw CBDA may also add support. Omega 3 ALA in addition to marine omega 3 EPA and DHA may enhance benefits. Additional omega 3 EPA would be recommended.

DERMATITIS, ATOPIC

Atopic dermatitis like eczema is a common chronic skin condition that causes inflammation and irritation. Atopic dermatitis is commonly seen in babies and young children although it can affect adults.

Symptoms

This skin condition appears as red, inflamed, dry, and itchy skin. You may experience other symptoms, such as:

- Blisters
- Crusting of skin
- Cracking of skin
- Scaling

Triggers

Triggers that may exacerbate or cause atopic dermatitis include weather (low humidity or cold temperatures), seasonal allergies, and the use of harsh soaps and detergents.

Conventional Treatment/Side Effects

The treatment for this skin condition usually involves the use of moisturizers (petroleum jelly and topical steroids).

Benefits of CBD

CBD's properties feature an anti-inflammatory agent that aids in relieving itching and dry, red skin.

How to Use

Use 3 to 30 mg CBD until symptoms are relieved. Be sure to decrease the amount of CBD with any worsening of symptoms. Omega 3 ALA, in addition to marine omega 3 EPA and DHA, may enhance benefits.

See also ECZEMA.

ECZEMA

Eczema is a description for a group of skin diseases that cause skin inflammation and irritation. There are about 11 different types of skin conditions that produce eczema. Atopic dermatitis is the most common type of eczema. Eczema is chronic and tends to flare up periodically and then subside.

Eczema affects about 10 to 20 percent of infants and about 3 percent of adults and children in the US. No cure has been found for the condition.

Symptoms

Eczema most often begins before the age of five and may persist into adolescence and adulthood. For some people, it flares periodically and then clears up for a time, even for several years. The following are symptoms that are associated with eczema and the damage it can cause:

- Itching, especially at night
- Raw, sensitive, swollen skin from scratching
- Red to brownish-gray patches
- Small, raised bumps, which may leak fluid and crust over when scratched
- Thickened, cracked, dry, scaly skin

Triggers

Factors that can worsen eczema signs and symptoms include:

- Bacteria and viruses
- Dry skin from long, hot baths and showers
- Dust and pollen
- Eggs, milk, peanuts, soybeans, fish, and wheat, in infants and children
- Heat and humidity changes
- Solvents, cleaners, soaps, and detergent
- Stress
- Sweating
- Tobacco smoke and air pollution
- Wool clothing, blankets, and carpets

Conventional Treatment/Side Effects

Since a cure for eczema has not yet been found, the first line of approach by most general practitioners and dermatologists is to prescribe topical corticosteroids. These are steroids that are applied in a cream or gel base to the areas of eczema on the skin. Some people have an allergic response to the steroids themselves, which can result in itching, white bumps, and a rash that resembles acne. Eczema can also become tolerant to steroids and reappear despite continued application.

Some of the following side effects can also be associated with the use of corticosteroid cream:

- Impaired wound healing   - Skin thinning
- Secondary infection

In addition to the use of corticosteroids, other conventional methods of treating eczema include: topical calcineurin inhibitors, as well as antibiotics, antifungals, anti-histamines, antivirals, and emollients. However, no conventional treatments offer permanent resolutions and have far more limitations and side effects than alternative methods and treatments.

Benefits of CBD

Fatty acids in omega-6 and omega-3 help maintain good skin health by keeping cell membranes flexible. In 2005, the *Journal of Dermatology Treatment* published a study done by Dr. J. Callaway on the treatment of eczema. Dr. Callaway found that the symptoms of skin dryness and itching significantly improved in patients suffering from eczema after using CBD for 20 weeks. He stated, "We saw remarkable reduction in dryness, itching, and an overall improvement in symptoms."

How to Use

Dr. Callaway discovered that 2 tablespoons of dietary CBD oil consumed daily can help relieve the effects of eczema. As the dosage of CBD differs for each person, it is best to start small and gradually increase until you experience the desired result. CBDA rich topical balms are reported to be effective in the treatment of eczema. Topical gold concentrates may also be required for treatment resistant cases. Isolated CBD crystals may produce topical products that are more drug like and corrective than natural daily use products. Use 3 to 15 mg of CBD twice daily for internal inflammation. Omega 3 ALA in addition to marine omega 3 EPA and DHA may enhance benefits.

EPILEPSY

Epilepsy is a chronic neurological disorder that is characterized by recurrent, unprovoked episodes of convulsions, known as seizures, or loss of consciousness. It can affect people of all ages. There are many types of seizures, which are typically classified by physicians as either generalized, focal, or unknown. Seizures usually last from a few seconds to a few minutes.

Symptoms

Seizures usually occur without warning. The symptoms may vary depending on the type. Usually, someone suffering from seizures will experience the same kind of seizure each time. Therefore, the symptoms will appear similar for each episode. The signs and symptoms may include:

- Changes in sensations (waves of heat or cold)
- Dazed behavior
- Heart racing
- Loss of awareness
- Loss of consciousness
- Muscles jerk out of control or twitch (arms and legs)
- Temporary confusion
- Weakening of muscles

Triggers

What causes the disorder may differ by the age of the person. If no clear cause is apparent, it may be a genetic factor. Common triggers of epileptic seizures may include:

Infants and Children

- Born with brain malformations
- Congenital disorders
- Drug use by mother
- Fever
- Head trauma

- Infections
- Intracranial hemorrhage

- Lack of oxygen during birth

Adults

- Alzheimer's disease
- Head injuries
- Stroke

- Trauma
- Tumors

Conventional Treatment/Side Effects

A large number of epileptic seizures are controlled by anticonvulsant drugs. The choice of anticonvulsant drug prescribed will depend on the person's age, overall health, and medical history. Although the drugs can control the seizures, they don't cure the disorder and most often people will need to continue taking the medication. Use of the drugs may result in adverse side effects, such as dizziness, fatigue, nausea, vomiting, rash, depression, and loss of appetite.

Benefits of CBD

Evidence from studies demonstrates that CBD could potentially be helpful in controlling seizures. The research has shown that CBD can act as an anticonvulsant and may even have antipsychotic effects. A number of studies have shown the use of CBD to be an effective method of reducing the number of seizures a person with epilepsy experiences.

One such study is that of Dr. Anup Patel, of Nationwide Children's Hospital and The Ohio State University College of Medicine in Columbus, who found that cannabidiol is an effective treatment for Lennox-Gastaut syndrome, a serious form of epilepsy. A group of 225 young patients with Lennox-Gastaut syndrome were tested. Each day, patients were administered either a higher or lower dose of cannabidiol, or an inactive placebo. The patients who took the higher dose experienced a 42 percent reduction in drop seizures overall. Furthermore, 40 percent of patients in that group saw that the amount of seizures they usually experienced was reduced by half or more. The patients who took the lower dose had a 37 percent reduction in drop seizures (atonic seizures) overall, with 36 percent experiencing less than half the usual amount of seizures. In contrast, those in the placebo group had a 17 percent reduction in drop seizures overall, with 15 percent seeing that their seizures were reduced by half or more.

More research needs to be completed to study the safety and efficacy of CBD; however the medical community is beginning to recognize the positive outcomes that some people have experienced from CBD rich extracts.

How to Use

Recommended dose is 30 mg. Self-medication is ill advised especially when taking multiple anti-epileptic medications. The drug-to-drug interactions with CBD in this patient population requires very strict medical monitoring, supervision, and care. Reports of miraculous cures are followed up years later to reveal another wall of treatment resistance has been hit and that the miracle cannabis strain no longer works. Hearts are broken, the promise of CBD is no longer kept, it fails to deliver. What suddenly changed? Our ECS (endocannabinoid system) changed, especially when we are very sick. The ECS may be our master control system, yet we never learn how to fully control it, and it may even do harm while attempting to heal.

FDA-approved CBD drugs are being developed for treatment resistant seizures that have no commercial counterpart or generics in the market today. These FDA-approved CBD drugs are not hemp extracts and will only be available at pharmacies. When treating epilepsy with CBD, the only product to ever be used must be filled at a pharmacy with a childproof cap. It is not recommended to use CBD sold on line or independent natural retailers.

EYE DISORDERS

See AGE-RELATED MACULAR DEGENERATION; GLAUCOMA.

FIBROMYALGIA

Fibromyalgia (FM) is a common condition that is characterized by chronic pain and tenderness in the muscles and bones, as well as fatigue. It mostly affects women, although men and children can also suffer from the condition. It can be a difficult disorder to diagnose because the main symptoms may be similar to symptoms of other conditions.

Symptoms

Pain is the main symptom and felt at different degrees at different times of the day. For some the pain is at its worse when they awake and improves as the day progresses. Different people may experience this pain in various ways, such as chronic, all-over, shooting, tender, aching and deep pain. Other common symptoms associated with FM may be:

- Anxiety
- Chronic fatigue
- Cognitive problems ("fibro fog")
- Depression
- Irritable bowel symptoms
- Migraines
- Restless leg
- Trouble sleeping

Triggers

Doctors aren't able to find a direct link related to FM, however a combination of factors may play a role in triggering the condition, including:

- Emotional trauma
- Family history
- Genetics
- Infections
- Physical trauma
- Sex (diagnosed more often in women)

Conventional Treatment/Side Effects

Commonly a healthcare provider will recommend medication or therapy to help reduce the symptoms associated with fibromyalgia. The common choices of medication are over-the-counter pain relievers, such as acetaminophen, ibuprofen, or naproxen sodium and antidepressants, such as Cymbalta. A prescription drug, such as tramadol, may also be recommended for pain relief.

Besides medications, a number of therapies (traditional and alternative) may be suggested to decrease the effects of the condition on your body. These include physical therapy, occupational therapy, acupuncture, yoga, or tai chi.

Over-the-counter medications, like all drugs, can cause side effects and may not be safe for everyone. The side effects generally include stomach upset or pain, nausea, diarrhea, or heartburn. In some cases, it may raise blood pressure, result in stomach ulcers or bleeding, or cause allergic reactions.

Benefits of CBD

Although there is a lack of scientific research, some recent reports have shown that people suffering from fibromyalgia have managed a number of symptoms with CBD oil. These reports cite that these patients were able to find relief from chronic pain, anxiety, depression, mood swings, and difficulty sleeping without the side effects of traditional drugs.

How to Use

As recommended by the CBD Oil Review, to treat chronic pain take 3 to 30 mg CBD by mouth for an average of 25 days. As serving size or dosage of CBD differs for each person, it is suggested to start small and gradually increase until you experience the desired result. Topical balms may also offer relief from pain, inflammation, and swelling. Omega 3 ALA in addition to marine omega 3 EPA and DHA may enhance benefits.

FM

See **FIBROMYALGIA.**

GLAUCOMA

Glaucoma is indicated when there has been damage to the optic nerve of the eye. It is the leading cause of blindness in people over the age of 60 years old. There are two types of glaucoma: primary open-angle, which is the most common, and closed-angle or narrow-angle.

Symptoms

In the early stages of open-angle glaucoma, there aren't any obvious signs or symptoms. On the other hand, symptoms for an attack of closed-angle glaucoma may include:

- Appearance of rainbows or halos
- Decreased vision
- Eye pain or pain in forehead
- Eye redness
- Hazy or blurred vision
- Headache
- Nausea
- Tunnel vision
- Vomiting

Triggers

Glaucoma occurs when fluid builds up in the front part of your eye. That extra fluid increases the pressure in your eye, damaging the optic nerve and causing vision loss. The reason for the buildup may include:

- Blocked blood vessels in the eye
- Eye infections (severe)
- Genetics
- Inflammation
- Injury to the eye, blunt or chemical

Conventional Treatment/Side Effects

Glaucoma is most commonly treated with eye drops. Although these eye drops decrease pressure by helping the fluid drain, they may cause some side effects, such as stinging or itching, dry mouth, blurred vision, and changes in energy level, heartbeat, and pulse.

An oral medication, usually a carbonic anhydrase inhibitor, may be prescribed as well if the eye drops don't decrease the pressure. Side effects include depression, upset stomach, kidney stones, frequent urination, and a tingling sensation in the toes and fingers. If the oral medication or eye drops fail to improve the patient's condition, surgery (laser or traditional) may be necessary.

Benefits of CBD

Animal studies have shown that CBD has been proven to be beneficial in decreasing intraocular pressure. One study, cited in *Graefe's Archive for Clinical and Experimental Ophthalmology* in 2000, stated that "applied cannabinoids directly to the eyes of rabbits recorded decreased intraocular pressure within 1.5 hours of administration and the effects lasted for more than 6 hours. In addition, the eye to which the cannabinoid had not been administered also experienced a decrease in intraocular pressure, but the effect lasted for 4 hours."

Scientific research submitted to the *European Journal of Neuroscience* found that "applying a cannabinoid directly to the human eye decreased intraocular pressure within 30 minutes and reached maximal reduction in the first 60 minutes." These studies, as well as other observations conducted, confirm that cannabinoids may decrease the intraocular pressure in the eye when administered topically or systemically.

How to Use

The recommended treatment for glaucoma is a single CBD dose of 15 to 30 mg. Omega 3 ALA in addition to marine omega 3 EPA and DHA may enhance benefits.

HEADACHE

Many people experience headaches at some point in their life. They can range from mild to very severe and can negatively impact anyone. The severity and the location of the pain are associated with the type of headache, such as tension headaches, cluster headaches, sinus headaches, rebound headaches, and migraine headaches.

Symptoms

The following signs or symptoms are characteristic of each kind of headache:

- Cluster headache: (occurs in groups) severe pain on one side of head, watery eye and nasal congestion or runny nose on that same side

- Migraine headaches: one sided, throbbing pain with a sensitivity to light and that may be accompanied by nausea and/or vomiting

- Rebound headaches: dull, tension-type headache or a more severe migraine-like headache

- Sinus headache: pain and pressure in sinuses and may be accompanied by fever

- Tension headache (most common): mild, moderate, or intense pain or pressure around the temples or back of head or neck

Triggers

Headaches are primarily caused by an inflammation of the blood vessels in and around the brain and/or the chemical activity in your brain. Triggers may be lifestyle factors and/ or a concealed disease, including:

- Alcohol
- Changes in waking/ sleeping patterns
- Dehydration
- Food additives
- Hormonal changes in women
- Infections

- Lack of exercise
- Medication overuse (rebound headache)
- Personality traits
- Skipping meals
- Sleep deprivation
- Stress

Conventional Treatment/Side Effects

Traditional headache treatment depends on the type of headache you're fighting. Tension headaches may be treated with over-the-counter pain killers, such as aspirin, ibuprofen and acetaminophen. The same over-the-counter medications may help to relieve pain from a migraine, although certain prescription medications also exist, such as Imitrex or Zomig.

Cluster headaches usually require injectable prescribed medications (for example, Imitrex and Sumavel) or prescribed nasal sprays (Zomig or Imitrex) which provide quick relief. The over-the-counter pain killers or nasal decongestants may help relieve pain from sinus headaches.

Although you may experience relief from headache pain, these common drugs may trigger nausea, sleepiness, fatigue, or a racing heartbeat. Use of these medications over a long period of time may result in rebound headaches.

Benefits of CBD

CBD products exhibit the ability to treat headaches and migraines. Studies have indicated a relationship between migraines and endocannabinoid dysfunction. In a survey conducted by SFGate, 100 percent of the population reported that CBD oil relieved their migraines.

At the University of Perugia in 2007, researchers found that the endocannabinoid levels in the cerebrospinal fluid of patients suffering from chronic migraines were quite low, inferring that an impairment of the endocannabinoid system might result in chronic head pain. Neurologist and cannabinoid researcher Dr. Ethan Russo took the relationship between endocannabinoid deficiency and migraines to develop the Clinical Endocannabinoid Theory. According to Dr. Russo's theory, plant-based cannabinoids like CBD can help restore balance to the endocannabinoid system.

How to Use

Using 15 mg to 30 mg of CBD twice daily is recommended. Vaping has also been reported to be an effective way to deliver fast relief with CBD. Omega 3 ALA in addition to marine omega 3 EPA and DHA may enhance benefits.

HEART DISEASE

Heart disease, or cardiovascular disease, is the leading cause of death in the United States and currently affects over 80 million Americans. It refers to any condition that affects the heart and blood vessels. Coronary artery disease, angina pectoris, atherosclerosis, congestive heart failure, and heart arrhythmias are among the most common cardiovascular conditions.

Symptoms

Symptoms of heart disease are generally caused by narrowed blood vessels or an abnormal heartbeat. People are often not aware that they have a heart condition until an emergency such as a heart attack or heart failure occurs. Common symptoms include:

- Bradycardia (slow heartbeat)
- Chest pain (angina)
- Dizziness
- Fainting
- Lightheadedness
- Pain in neck, jaw, throat, or back
- Pain or numbness in legs or arms
- Shortness of breath
- Tachycardia (racing heart)

Triggers

Along with genetics, which is a significant contributor, other common factors that can cause heart disease include:

- Chronic stress
- Diabetes
- Excessive alcohol/drug use
- High blood pressure
- High cholesterol
- Obesity
- Physical inactivity
- Poor diet
- Smoking

Conventional Treatment/Side Effects

Diagnosis and treatment of various heart conditions will vary. Along with suggesting lifestyle changes, such as eating a healthy low-fat diet and incorporating a moderate exercise program, physicians may also recommend medication. Included among the most commonly prescribed conventional medications for heart disease are ACE inhibitors to widen arteries, vasodilators to allow easier blood flow through the vessels, and blood thinners to prevent the formation of clots.

The possible side effects of ACE inhibitors may include dizziness, fatigue, and rapid heartbeat. Common side effects associated with vasodilators are edema (fluid retention), heart palpitations, joint and chest pain, headaches, and nausea. Blood thinners increase the risk of bleeding, which can be life-threatening. Do not take blood thinners if you have a bleeding disorder like hemophilia, stomach or intestinal bleeding, an ulcer, or very high blood pressure. Avoid them if you have had recent or upcoming surgery or dental work; a recent head injury or aneurysm; or severe heart disease. Pregnant women should avoid blood thinners as they have been linked to birth defects.

Many drugs can have serious interactions when taken with warfarin or heparin. Before taking any blood thinner, be sure to inform your doctor about any and all medications you are currently taking or have used recently. Any type of heart medication should always be taken under the watchful eye of a doctor or other healthcare professional.

Benefits of CBD

CBD oil could prove to be very helpful in treating heart disease. Because of its anti-inflammatory properties, CBD can help relax the blood vessels, allowing blood to flow through more easily. It has shown positive effects in patients with ischemia, or an insufficient supply of blood to the heart muscles. CBD has proven effective in patients who have heart disease caused by diabetes and stroke. It reduces the cardiovascular response to stress and has a direct effect on the longevity of white blood cells.

A 2013 article issued in the *British Journal of Clinical Pharmacology* produced data that showed the positive role CBD plays in the treatment of heart disease. CBD is known to reduce tension on blood vessel walls. *In vivo* CBD treatments in the heart have been shown to reduce the amount of dead tissue created by lack of blood supply, known as infarct. As cited in a recent study published in the *Journal of Agricultural and Food Chemistry*, CBD oil contains a high concentration of sterols that may help reduce risk of heart disease and promote heart health.

How to Use

Recommended dosage is 3 to 30 mg of CBD taken daily. Check with your healthcare provider before taking CBD.

HIGH BLOOD PRESSURE

High blood pressure, or hypertension, affects nearly 30 percent of people in the US alone. Involving the force of blood flow, hypertension can damage arteries and lead to life-threatening conditions like heart disease and stroke. A blood pressure reading is shown as two numbers—a top number, which shows the force of blood flow when the heart is beating (systolic pressure); and a lower number, which shows the force when the heart is resting (diastolic pressure).

According to the current recommendations of the American Heart Association, a reading under 120/80 is considered normal, while a reading of 140/90 or above is considered high.

One frightening aspect of hypertension is that it doesn't exhibit any obvious symptoms. Because of this, many people are unaware that they have it, which is why it is sometimes called "the silent killer." High blood pressure cannot be cured, but it can be managed successfully.

Symptoms

Typically, high blood pressure does not exhibit any unusual symptoms. The only way to know for certain if you have it is to have your physician take a reading. Some common inconclusive symptoms can include:

- Blood spots on the eyes
- Chest pains
- Facial flushing
- Fatigue
- Nosebleeds
- Severe headaches
- Shortness of breath

Triggers

Common factors that can cause high blood pressure include:

- Age (older people are more likely to develop high blood pressure)
- Genetics/family history
- Excessive alcohol use
- High sodium/low potassium diet
- Obesity
- Physical inactivity
- Smoking
- Stress

Conventional Treatment/Side Effects

To treat high blood pressure, doctors will often first suggest making some basic lifestyle changes, such as eating a healthy low-sodium diet and exercising regularly. Quitting smoking and reducing or eliminating alcohol use can also help to reduce high blood pressure.

The most common recommended medications include diuretics, or water pills. Diuretics help reduce blood volume by eliminating excess sodium and water from the body. Beta blockers, which often work in combination with other drugs, are prescribed to help open blood vessels and reduce pressure on the heart. Angiotensin II receptor blockers (ARBs) and calcium channel blockers help relax blood vessels to allow easier blood flow.

Beta blockers may cause drowsiness, dizziness, dry mouth, and constipation or diarrhea. Fatigue, headaches, dizziness, and dry cough are common reactions to ARBs. Calcium channel blockers may cause lightheadedness, constipation, swelling of feet and ankles, and increased appetite. Grapefruit and grapefruit juice interacts negatively with calcium channel blockers and must be avoided. Alcohol should also be avoided as it interferes with the drug's positive effects while increasing its side effects.

Benefits of CBD

Recent research suggests that the body's cannabinoid system plays a significant role in controlling blood pressure. Animal studies have demonstrated that endocannabinoids suppress hypertension and reduce blood pressure.

In a study originally published in 2015, Christopher Stanley and his team at the University of Nottingham School of Medicine set out to discover if endocannabinoids could be the future replacement for today's commonly used high blood pressure drugs. The aim of the study was to determine the effects of CBD on blood vessels. The results of this study brought further insight into CBD's impact on the body's internal endocannabinoid system: the endocannabinoid receptors proved to play a vital role blood vessel constriction and relaxation. In a constricted vessel, activation of CB1 receptors with CBD caused the vessels to relax and dilate, thus lowering blood pressure.

In an article cited in the *British Journal of Clinical Pharmacology* in 2012, evidence suggested that CBD is beneficial in the workings of the cardiovascular system. The animal study showed that CBD protects against the vascular damage caused by a high glucose environment, inflammation, and type 2 diabetes, as well as aids in the vascular permeability (the ability of a blood vessel wall to allow the flow of small molecules and whole cells) associated with such environments.

How to Use

Recommended dosage is 3 to 30 mg of CBD taken twice daily. If you are taking medication for blood pressure, you should consult your physician before taking CBD.

INFLAMMATION

Inflammation is the immune system's attempt to heal the body after an injury, defend it against foreign invaders like viruses and bacteria, and repair damaged tissue. During this process, the body's white blood cells are released into the bloodstream and travel to the affected area, where they (along with hormones and nutrients) attack the harmful invaders and begin the healing process.

Inflammation can be acute or chronic and can occur internally or externally. *Acute inflammation* is short-term and activated by such injuries as a cut on the skin, a sprained ankle, or a stubbed toe; as well as a bacterial or viral infection. The inflammatory process involves increased blood flow to the affected area, and often results in swelling, warmth, redness, and pain.

Chronic inflammation is long-term. It can result from failure to eliminate the cause of an acute inflammation, or it can be from a persistent, unresolved low-intensity irritant. Often, chronic inflammation is caused by a faulty autoimmune response that attacks healthy tissue, mistaking it as harmful.

Asthma, rheumatoid arthritis, and ulcerative colitis are just a few of the hundreds of autoimmune disorders, and nearly all include inflammation as one of the symptoms. Chronic inflammation has also been implicated as a contributor to such serious illnesses as heart disease, stroke, and certain cancers.

Symptoms

The acronym PRISH refers to the five most significant symptoms of acute inflammation: Pain, Redness, Immobility (loss of joint function), Swelling, and Heat. For chronic inflammation, the symptoms are not always as apparent. They usually occur when the associated disease or health condition presents itself. Some of the more common symptoms have included constant or ongoing:

- Depression
- Fatigue
- Joint or muscle pain
- Stomach/gastrointestinal pain

Triggers

Typically, the symptom of a broader disease or condition (often in the gut), chronic inflammation may be triggered by:

- Allergies, food and environmental
- Autoimmune disorders
- Digestive issues
- Environmental toxins (heavy metals)
- Hormone imbalance
- Obesity
- Poor diet (processed, sugary, fast foods)
- Sleep deprivation
- Stress, emotional and physical

Conventional Treatment/Side Effects

Symptoms of acute inflammation are often treated with over-the-counter nonsteroidal anti-inflammatory drugs (NSAIDs), such as aspirin and ibuprofen. These drugs, however, are associated with a number of possible side effects, including dizziness, stomach pain, ringing in the ears, high blood pressure, and the onset of stomach ulcers.

Corticosteroids, such as prednisone, may be prescribed to treat a number of inflammatory diseases and conditions. Taken orally, by injection, or applied topically, corticosteroids can be effective, but they also carry the risk of serious side effects. High blood pressure, edema (fluid retention), osteoporosis, cataracts, weight gain, and memory issues are among the most common.

Benefits of CBD

Ongoing research indicates that CBD oil may be effective in treating inflammatory conditions without the serious side effects and health complications affiliated with conventional treatments.

A 2006 study that appeared in the *European Journal of Pharmacology* set out to determine the effect of cannabidiol as an effective treatment in managing chronic inflammatory and neuropathic (nerve) pain in laboratory rats. After pain was induced in the study subjects, they were given oral doses of CBD. After seven days of repeated treatment, the subjects showed a reduction in pain and inflammation. The results indicated that CBD may indirectly affect the cannabinoid receptors in the brain—CB1 and CB2—that help to manage pain.

Results of a study done at the University of Mississippi Medical Center and published in the *Free Radical Biology & Medicine Journal* showed that cannabidiol can be helpful in reducing the impact of inflammation on oxidative stress. Oxidative stress and inflammation are known contributors to a number of conditions, including high blood pressure, rheumatoid arthritis, Type 1 and Type 2 diabetes, atherosclerosis, depression, and Alzheimer's disease.

How to Use

Recommended dosage is 3 to 45 mg. Combine CBDA and CBD with THC for those who can tolerate THC. Never self-medicate with THC. Make sure you are guided by a qualified physician. Topical balms and concentrates may be effective for inflammatory conditions of the skin. Omega 3 ALA in addition to marine omega 3 EPA and DHA may enhance benefits.

Depending on the dosage and the person, CBD can be stimulating if taken prior to sleep, while some people report dramatic improvements in sleep quality. The best way to determine if the extracts will help you fall and stay asleep is to slowly titrate with drops or sprays, gradually increasing the dose to achieve the desired effect.

Some people find it more beneficial to start the day with CBD due to its effects on the neurotransmitter serotonin, while other report best results one hour prior to bed time. Omega 3 ALA in addition to marine omega 3 EPA and DHA may enhance benefits.

INSOMNIA

A common sleep disorder, insomnia is characterized by the inability to fall asleep, to stay asleep, and/or to fall back asleep. The average adult needs between seven to eight hours of sleep per night; insomniacs sleep much less than that.

Short-term (acute) insomnia can last a few days or weeks, while long-term (chronic) insomnia can stretch for months or even longer. Insomnia is considered chronic if it lasts at least three nights a week for a month or more.

Sleep is an important aspect of good health both mentally and physically. Typically, people who suffer from insomnia do not perform optimally at work or school; their reaction time while driving and performing tasks is compromised; and they have a greater risk of serious health conditions like high blood pressure and heart disease.

Symptoms

Common daytime symptoms of those with insomnia include:

■ Anxiety   ■ Depression

- Difficulty concentrating
- Emotional outbursts
- Fatigue
- Headaches
- Irritability
- Lack of energy
- Lack of interest in social functions
- Mood swings
- Sleepiness

Triggers

An irregular or interrupted sleep schedule is a common cause of insomnia and may affect people who travel often or who work alternating day and night shifts. Other likely causes include:

- Alcohol, caffeine, nicotine
- Certain medical conditions, like acid reflux, asthma
- Change in environment
- Chronic pain
- Eating late at night
- Irregular bedtimes
- Sleep-related disorders like sleep apnea and restless leg syndrome
- Stress/anxiety
- Uncomfortable sleep environment
- Using electronics before bed

Conventional Treatment/Side Effects

Treatment for insomnia can be as simple as changing one's bedtime habits—going to sleep earlier or later than usual or turning off TVs and electronic devices an hour or so before bedtime. If insomnia is caused by stress, relaxation and deep-breathing techniques as well as yoga may help. In some cases, over-the-counter medications like antihistamines are recommended, but they are not without side effects. Along with drowsiness, antihistamines may cause blurred vision and dry mouth. For more severe cases of insomnia, prescription medications—sedatives, tranquilizers, anti-anxiety drugs—may be prescribed.

Depending on the type of drug and dosage, sleep aids can become habit-forming and are capable of producing serious side effects. These may include extreme agitation; personality changes; hallucinations; and symptoms of depression, including thoughts of suicide. Performing an activity while asleep—driving, eating, talking on the phone—and having no recollection of the activity upon waking up are also common. Prescription sleep aids may also interact with other medications, vitamins, and herbal supplements. Before taking any medication, be sure to discuss the possible side effects and drug interactions with your healthcare provider.

Benefits of CBD

As an anti-anxiety aid, CBD can be effective in relieving insomnia-causing stress and regulating sleep schedules. According to Project CBD—a nonprofit organization whose mission is to provide the most current, accurate information on the medicinal properties of cannabidiol—CBD activates certain receptors in the brain that result in "a balancing effect that facilitates a good night's sleep."

One recent study published in the *Journal of Psychopharmacology* assessed the effects of CBD on the sleep-wake cycle of laboratory rats. The subjects were distributed into four groups, with three groups given injections of CBD in doses of 2.5 mg/kg, 10 mg/kg, and 40 mg/kg. The fourth group was given a placebo. Sleep recordings of the subjects were made for four days. The first two days involved baseline recordings. On the third day (test day), the subjects were given the CBD injections. They were also recorded the day after the test. On test day, the two groups given 10 and 40 mg/kg CBD showed a significant increase in the total percentage of sleep during the light period of the day compared to the placebo group. The group injected with 40 mg/kg also showed an increase in REM sleep latency, with a significant decrease on the day following the test. (Sleep latency is the amount of time it takes to transition from wakefulness to sleep. A lower sleep latency score indicates sleep deprivation.) From this study, the researchers concluded that the administration of CBD appears to have an effect in increasing both total sleep time and sleep latency on the day of administration.

A case study that appeared in a recent edition of *The Permanente Journal* involved a ten-year-old girl with post-traumatic stress disorder (PTSD). After experiencing a traumatizing event at age three, the subject was largely neglected by her parents, and eventually placed in the custody of her grandmother. Psychotherapy began at age seven. Along with low self-esteem and a variety of behavioral issues, she experienced anxiety and restless, interrupted sleep. Initially. She had been prescribed a variety of medications, vitamins, and supplements for various issues. At age ten, she was given CBD oil to treat her insomnia and reduce anxiety. She was given a 25 mg dose at bedtime and sublingual spray (6 mg to 12 mg) during the day as needed for anxiety. She experienced a gradual increase in the quality and quantity of her sleep and a notable decrease in anxiety. After five months, she was sleeping through most nights and experiencing no side effects from the CBD oil.

How to Use

Take 3 mg to 30 mgs at bedtime.

IRRITABLE BOWEL SYNDROME

An estimated 35 million Americans suffer from irritable bowel syndrome (IBS)—a chronic gastrointestinal condition in which the intestines do not function properly. Normally, waste moves through the intestines and is eliminated from the body thanks to the rhythmic muscular contractions of the intestines.

With IBS, the contractions are irregular and erratic—either too strong or not strong enough. This results in a number of uncomfortable, often severe symptoms that typically include abdominal pain, cramping, bloating, and diarrhea and/or constipation.

In many cases, the gastrointestinal tract is sensitive to certain dietary influences, which further complicates the condition. Unlike Crohn's disease and ulcerative colitis, which are serious inflammatory bowel diseases, IBS is considered a functional problem of the intestines.

There is no specific test for diagnosing IBS. The condition is generally diagnosed by eliminating more serious problems, such as diverticulitis, ulcerative colitis, and colorectal cancer, which can produce symptoms that are similar to IBS. Its diagnosis is also based on the duration and frequency of the symptoms, which occur at least three times a month for at least six months.

Symptoms

The signs and symptoms of IBS, as well as their severity, will vary. Typically, they occur after eating, and include:

- Abdominal pain
- Bloating
- Cramping
- Diarrhea and/or constipation
- Gas
- Loss of appetite
- Mucus in the stool
- Nausea
- Painful bowel movements

Triggers

Although the cause of this condition is unknown, the following factors have been known to trigger or worsen the attacks:

- Anxiety
- Artificial sweeteners
- Caffeinated, carbonated, and alcoholic beverages
- Food sensitivities (often gluten)
- Lactose intolerance
- Overgrowth of intestinal bacteria
- Stress

Conventional Treatment/Side Effects

Dietary modifications are typically the first recommendation for those with IBS. Avoiding trigger foods and maintaining a high-fiber diet based on vegetables and whole grains can help reduce or prevent an IBS flare up. If the problem persists, medication may be suggested.

The doctor may recommend an anti-diarrheal like loperimide (Imodium), which slows the movement of the digestive tract, allowing more time for the reabsorption of water from the stool. This type of medication does not reduce the pain or bloating associated with the diarrhea, and it can cause dizziness, dry mouth, and fatigue. In some people, it can initiate severe constipation, nausea, and irregular heartbeat.

To help prevent bowel spasms, medications such as dicyclomine (Bentyl) and hyoscyamine (Levsin) may be prescribed. However, they must be taken with caution as they can make urinating difficult and worsen constipation.

For those with constipation, a laxative may help treat the symptoms, but not necessarily the pain.

Benefits of CBD

In addition to producing a calming effect in patients, CBD works as a powerful anti-spasmodic, which helps relieve the pain associated with irritable bowel syndrome. Recent research has shown that cannabinoids play a crucial role in controlling gastrointestinal inflammation and motility. According to an abstract that appeared in *European Review for Medical and Pharmacological Sciences*, "Consistently, in vivo studies have shown that cannabinoids reduce gastrointestinal transit in rodents through activation of CB1 receptors. . . . Cannabinoids also reduce gastrointestinal motility in randomized clinical trials."

Many people with IBS suffer from anxiety and depression. While the psychoactive THC component of the cannabis plant has been shown to raise mental spirits, a 2016 study showed the same results with CBD—the plant's non psychoactive component. Minutes after the study's rodent subjects were given a single dose of CBD, they displayed signs of reduced anti-social and anxiety-like behavior.

An article in the May 2013 issue of *Phytotherapy Research* cited CBD as "a promising drug for the therapy of inflammatory bowel diseases." CBD is continuously touted for its anti-inflammatory properties and shows great potential as a treatment for IBD and other gut disturbances.

How to Use

Take 10 to 15 mg of CBD daily. Taking 15 mg of gold soft-gels have also been reported to be effective. THC may be helpful if the patient can tolerate it and is under a physician's care. Excessive oils may not be tolerated, so look for ultra-high omega 3 EPA and DHA to support the ECS and the inflammatory response.

MACULAR DEGENERATION

See **AGE-RELATED MACULAR DEGENERATION.**

MENOPAUSE

See **HORMONAL IMBALANCE.**

MIGRAINE HEADACHE

See **HEADACHE.**

MS

See **MULTIPLE SCLEROSIS.**

MULTIPLE SCLEROSIS

Multiple sclerosis (MS) is a disease of the central nervous system in which the immune system attacks nerve fibers in the body. The breakdown of the protective nerve fiber sheath causes miscommunications between your brain and the rest of your body, damages nerves, and can potentially disable the spinal cord.

Symptoms

The symptoms of MS depend on how badly the nerves are damaged. Severe MS can cause a patient to lose the ability to walk, while patients with mild MS may only experience numbness. The most common symptoms, both mild and severe, are listed below:

- Bowel and bladder function problems
- Dizziness
- Fatigue
- Numbness or weakness (often occurring on one side of the body at a time)
- Paralysis
- Partial or complete vision loss
- Shock-like sensations in the neck
- Slurred speech
- Tremor and a lack of coordination

Triggers

It is not known what causes MS, although it is classified as an autoimmune disease. Some of the possible risk factors are the following:

- Age (onset is typically between the ages of 15 and 60)

- Climate and environment (MS is more common in temperate-climate areas)

- Gender (women are twice as likely as men to develop MS)

- Genetics/family history

- Having certain autoimmune diseases

- Having certain infections, such as Epstein-Barr virus

- Race (white people have the highest rates of MS)

Conventional Treatment/Side Effects

Currently there are no effective medications or treatments for MS. Treatments are mainly given to ease the painful symptoms and make patients more comfortable, or to slow down the disease's progression. Such treatments include corticosteroids, taken orally or through an IV, which reduce inflammation in the nerves. Another treatment is plasma exchange, in which the plasma in your blood is separated from the blood cells. The blood cells are mixed with albumin, a protein solution, and then filtered back into your body.

Treatments to slow MS's progression include ocrelizumab, which is the only FDA-approved therapy for primary-progressive MS. Having primary-progressive MS means that the disease worsens from the onset, without relapses or remissions. Ocrelizumab is an antibody medication and has been shown in trials to impede the disability from becoming worse.

Patients with relapsing-remitting MS, meanwhile, experience intermittent attacks of neurological symptoms followed by periods of remission. Ocrelizumab can also be used to treat this form of MS as it has been shown to reduce the amount of relapses one experiences. Other treatments for this form of MS are beta interferons, which are injections that can reduce the severity of relapses. Glatiramer acetate, which is also injected and has been shown to block the immune system from attacking the nerve fibers and dimethyl fumarate, which is an oral medication, may reduce relapses.

Other therapies for MS include physical therapy to strengthen the weakened muscles and improve mobility; muscle relaxants; and anti-fatigue medications. The American Academy of Neurology recommends oral cannabis extract to treat symptoms of muscle spasticity and pain. Below, we will look more into the literature surrounding CBD's use in treating MS.

Benefits of CBD

Dozens of studies have been published illustrating the benefits of CBD on the symptoms of MS. Much of the research has been performed using Sativex, a medication that consists of THC and CBD in a 1:1 ratio. Sativex may become the first FDA-approved prescription marijuana extract.

In 2011, a drug profile for Sativex was published in the *Expert Review of Neurotherapeutics*. In the profile, the authors detailed what Sativex is (a 1:1 mix of THC and CBD available as an oromucosal spray) and its uses in various clinical trials. The article reported that the results from these clinical trials generally demonstrated "a reduction in the severity of the symptoms associated with spasticity." Spasticity is common in MS, involving muscles that stiffen and are difficult to move or control. Patients experienced a higher quality of life when they added Sativex to their treatment regimen. The profile concluded that "initial well-controlled studies with Sativex oromucosal spray administered as an add-on to usual therapy have produced promising results and highlight encouraging avenues for future research."

In a study published in 2013, Sativex was used to relieve symptoms of muscle spasticity. The fifteen-week-long double-blind, placebo-controlled trial involved 337 MS patients with spasticity. Results found that, compared with those who were treated with a placebo, 98 percent of patients treated with Sativex found some form of relief in the first four weeks of treatment. Any side effects from the Sativex dose were mild to moderate. The study's authors found that "Sativex treatment resulted in a significant reduction in treatment-resistant spasticity, in subjects with advanced MS and severe spasticity. The response observed within the first 4 weeks of treatment appears to be a useful aid to prediction of responder/ non-responder status."

One of the leading researchers in CBD research, Dr. Zvi Vogel of Israel, helped write a 2011 study that demonstrated how CBD helped mice with MS symptoms. The mice had a condition similar to MS, in which their limbs were partially paralyzed. After being injected with CBD, the mice began to move and walk around again without limping. The CBD-treated group of mice had significantly less inflammation in their spinal cords than the untreated group. The CBD worked by stopping the mice's immune cells from attacking nerve cells in their spinal cords.

The Israeli researchers followed up this study with another study in 2013. In this study, the researchers isolated harmful immune cells from paralyzed mice. These immune cells had been harming the brains and spinal cords of the mice. Using THC and CBD, the researchers found that both of these compounds helped reduce the number of inflammatory molecules being produced— in particular, an inflammatory molecule called interleukin 17 (IL-17), which is often indicated in MS cases. The study concluded that "the presence of CBD or THC restrains the immune cells from triggering the production of inflammatory molecules, and limits the molecules' ability to reach and damage the brain and spinal cord."

How to Use

The cannabinoid drug Satevix is a 1:1 ratio of CBD and THC extracted from marijuana and approved around the world for the treatment of multiple sclerosis (MS) Self-medication in this population is ill advised and not recommended. If approved by the FDA here in the United States, Sativex prescriptions for a tested ration of CBD and THC for MS would only be available in pharmacies. Omega 3 ALA in addition to marine omega 3 EPA and DHA may enhance benefits.

NAUSEA AND VOMITING

Nausea and vomiting are not diseases; however they are symptoms of a number of conditions. While nausea is commonly triggered by a "stomach flu," it may be a symptom of a number of serious conditions and illnesses.

Symptoms

Symptoms that occur with nausea and vomiting include:

- Abdominal pain
- Diarrhea
- Dry mouth
- Excessive sweating
- Fever
- Lightheadedness
- Rapid pulse
- Vertigo

Triggers

The following may cause nausea or vomiting:

- Bowel obstruction
- Early stages of pregnancy (nausea occurs in approximately 50 percent to 90 percent of all pregnancies; vomiting in 25 percent to 55 percent)
- Emotional stress (such as fear)
- Food poisoning
- Gallbladder disease
- Infections (such as the "stomach flu")
- Intense pain
- Medication-induced vomiting
- Motion sickness or seasickness
- Some forms of cancer

Conventional Treatment/Side Effects

Meclizine hydrochloride (Bonine) is an antihistamine that is effective in the treatment of nausea, vomiting, and dizziness associated with motion sickness. The more common side effects of meclizine hydrochloride can include drowsiness, headache, blurry vision, dry mouth, and tiredness.

Dramamine is an antiemetic, which means it prevents vomiting. It used to prevent and treat nausea. Drowsiness, constipation, dry mouth/nose/throat, and blurred vision are some of the possible side effects of Dramamine. Other medicines used as treatment include cyclizine, dimenhydrinate, diphenhydramine,

Benefits of CBD

Cannabidiol indirectly activates the receptor CB1 and other targets within the endocannabinoid system, thus regulating vomiting and nausea-like symptoms in a wide range of ailments. Research has proven it to be an effective antiemetic (anti-nausea/vomiting) treatment with fewer side effects than many drugs.

Advocates of CBD are hopeful that CBD oil will soon become a widely accepted treatment for nausea and vomiting inducing conditions and illnesses. However, it is crucial that one does not self-medicate without a proper diagnosis and determining the cause of the nausea and vomiting.

How to Use

The FDA approved cannabinoid drugs from the 1980s for nausea and vomiting extracts or the extended half-life and longer relief of ingestible dietary supplements or edibles. CBDA may offer an alternative to those who cannot tolerate THC, while some report that CBD is more effective. Due to the large distribution of serotonin receptors in the gut, too much CBDA may actually cause nausea. It's about fine tuning so proceed slowly. Recommended dosage is 3 to 30 mg of CBDA or CBD taken daily. Check with your healthcare provider.

OPIATE ADDICTION

See ADDICTION, OPIATE.

PANIC ATTACK

See ANXIETY DISORDERS.

PMS

See PREMENSTRUAL SYNDROME.

POST TRAUMATIC STRESS DISORDER

See ANXIETY DISORDERS.

PREMENSTRUAL SYNDROME

If you are female, you have likely experienced premenstrual syndrome (PMS) at least once in your lifetime. It is characterized by a number of symptoms that generally appear one to two weeks before a woman menstruates. Although not a disease itself, PMS can be a painful and unpleasant experience. The symptoms can last anywhere from a day or two up to a week.

Symptoms that appear to be severe PMS may actually be indicative of another condition, such as endometriosis. A more severe form of PMS is PMDD, or Premenstrual Dysphoric Disorder. If you are experiencing intense PMS-like symptoms, it is best to speak with a doctor to determine if these symptoms are part of another condition.

Symptoms

Symptoms mostly include changes in mood, although some changes in physical appearance are noted. More than 200 symptoms have been linked with PMS. General symptoms include:

- Abdominal cramps
- Acne
- Anxiety
- Bloating
- Change in libido
- Depression
- Fatigue
- Food cravings
- Headache
- Irritability
- Lower back pain
- Mood swing

Triggers

The exact cause of PMS is unknown, although it is likely caused by hormonal changes that occur during the menstrual cycle. Symptoms can be worsened, but not caused, by poor diet or a pre-existing mood disorder, such as major depression disorder. Other risk factors include:

- Age: Women in their twenties through early forties are more likely to experience symptoms.
- Family history of depression
- Having at least one child
- High stress level

Conventional Treatment/Side Effects

There is not a "cure-all" for PMS, but many treatments are used with varying results. Lifestyle changes, such as eating a diet high in vitamins and minerals and low in sodium and exercising, can help reduce bloating and improve mood. Specifically, foods high in the substance tryptophan—such as turkey, milk, and bananas—can be beneficial. Tryptophan helps to build the hormone serotonin and serotonin levels drop during PMS.

Medications that interact with hormones are sometimes used in more severe cases. For example, birth control pills may reduce symptoms in some women—but cause symptoms in other women. Antidepressant medications can be used in intervals to treat symptoms as they occur, although this may not be effective and can cause side effects.

Midol, an over-the-counter medication specifically targeting PMS symptoms (especially cramps), is a popular treatment. Other over-the-counter medications that are used to treat pain and cramps include aspirin and ibuprofen. At-home remedies can include using a heating pad to reduce cramps and pain; using essential oils such as lavender to reduce stress; and supplementing with calcium, magnesium, vitamin B6, and vitamin D.

Benefits of CBD

CBD may be useful in managing PMS. In an article for the website Goop, Dr. Julie Holland described how CBD could benefit women struggling with PMS. CBD has anti-inflammatory, anti-anxiety, and muscle-relaxant properties. To exercise these effects, CBD interacts with the molecules in the endocannabinoid system responsible for managing stress and pain.

The endocannabinoid system is made up of molecules that are similar to cannabis and help reduce stress and pain. The most significant of these molecules, anandamide, maintains balance in the hormonal and nervous systems. A higher anandamide level is linked with better stress management, according to Dr. Holland. Consuming CBD activates this endocannabinoid system to help bring the body back to a state of homeostasis.

The research focusing on PMS symptoms and cannabinoids has found that CBD "relaxes the mind and body" and "suppresses headaches and pain." In addition, the omega-6 and omega-3 fatty acids are essential fats that help to regulate blood sugar levels, "fluctuations which are related to PMS."

How to Use

Recommended dosage is 3 to 30 mg of CBD and/or a CBDA-rich topical balm preparation taken daily. Check with your personal healthcare provider. Omega 3 ALA in addition to marine omega 3 EPA and DHA may enhance benefits.

See also ANXIETY DISORDERS.

SCHIZOPHRENIA

Schizophrenia is a mental illness in which a person experiences a distorted reality. The inability to think clearly, irrational behavior, and wildly varying emotions are all indicative of schizophrenia.

Specifically, people with schizophrenia experience delusions, or thoughts that are not based in reality. They also often have visual or auditory hallucinations, especially hearing voices. Patients may be easily agitated or depressed, and may move and react oddly—for example, making excessive, useless movements. It is a critical, chronic condition that requires lifelong treatment to manage.

Symptoms

Schizophrenia symptoms can vary in their severity. In some patients, symptoms may always be present, while in others, symptoms get worse and then better. The disease usually starts to surface in your twenties. The following are the most common symptoms:

- Abnormal emotional responses
- Abnormal movements
- Delusions
- Disorganized thinking
- Hallucinations
- Hearing voices
- Loss of interest in hobbies
- Monotone speech
- Neglect of hygiene
- Social withdrawal
- Suicidal thoughts

Triggers

Although an exact cause has not been determined, schizophrenia is thought to be caused by a combination of genetics/family history, past psychoactive drug use, brain chemistry, and environment.

Conventional Treatment/Side Effects

In most cases, medication is necessary for managing schizophrenia. A class of drugs called anti-psychotics are most often prescribed. They work on the dopamine neurotransmitter in the brain, which is responsible for managing emotions, movements, and generating pleasure. There are two types of antipsychotics. First-generation antipsychotics are less expensive than second-generation antipsychotics, but tend to have more severe side effects, including the possibility of developing a movement disorder. Both classes of antipsychotics block similar receptors in the brain.

Therapy and interventions may be effective in conjunction with prescription medicine. Such therapies can include individual therapy to teach patients to recognize abnormal thoughts and warning signs of a relapse; family therapy to extend support to patients' loved ones; and social skills training. In addition, many people with schizophrenia require at-home aides or case managers to help them take care of themselves and/or become employed.

Benefits of CBD

High-THC cannabis can worsen symptoms of schizophrenia, especially anxiety and psychosis. CBD, on the other hand, cuts down thesey effects of THC.

A study published in the *Brazilian Journal of Medical and Biological Research* stated, "the antipsychotic-like properties of CBD have been investigated in animal models...which suggested that CBD has a pharmacological profile similar to atypical [second-generation] antipsychotic drugs."

According to a study conducted in the Illawarra Health and Medical Research Institute (IHMR), CBD "once isolated, could be used to treat negative cognitive symptoms of the severe mental illness—including social withdrawal and blunted emotional expression."

In another study led by Markus Leweke, University of Cologne in Germany, thirty-nine patients hospitalized for psychotic episodes were studied. Nineteen patients were treated with amisulpride, an antipsychotic medication, and the other twenty patients were given cannabidiol. Both groups showed a significant improvement in their symptoms at the end of the four-week trial. The patients taking CBD showed no difference from those taking amisulpride. Researchers concluded that CBD was not only on par with antipsychotic drugs in treating schizophrenia, but also free of the typical side effects associated with antipsychotics.

How to Use

Recommended dosage is 3 to 30 mg of CBD taken twice daily. Concentrated extracts may be most effective when combined with higher yamounts of omega 3 EPA and DHA.

SKIN CONDITIONS

See **ECZEMA.**

SLEEP DISORDERS

See **INSOMNIA.**

THROMBOSIS

See **BLOOD CLOTS.**

THYROID DISORDER

See **HORMONAL IMBALANCE.**

ULCERATIVE COLITIS

Ulcerative colitis is a long-term inflammatory bowel disease causing inflammation and ulcers (sores) in the rectum and colon. The condition can be painful, embarrassing, and debilitating. It can affect people of all ages.

Symptoms

Symptoms may present ythemselves differently and progress differently in each person, however common symptoms may be:

- Abdominal pain
- Bloody stools
- Constipation
- Diarrhea, persistent
- Fever
- Frequent/urgent bowel movements
- Loss of appetite
- Mucus in stools
- Muscle aches
- Weight loss

Anxiety and stress may cause the symptoms to worsen.

Triggers

Ulcerative colitis may begin gradually and may worsen over time. The exact cause is unknown, but studies have indicated that the following factors may play a role in the condition.

- Heredity
- Environmental factors
- Over-active immune system

Although stress and diet are not causes, research has shown that they may increase the chances of flare-ups.

Conventional Treatment/Side Effects

Depending on the severity of the condition, certain anti-inflammatory drugs may be prescribed, or surgery may be the option. Because some these drugs have severe side effects and because drugs that work for some may not work for others, it may take time to settle on a drug that helps you.

The drugs most commonly prescribed for this condition are aminosalicylates or corticosteroids. Antibiotics and immunosuppressant drugs may be prescribed as well. These drugs have a number of side effects, such as digestive distress, headaches, insomnia, and more serious side effects, for example high blood pressure, diabetes, osteoporosis, and a small risk of developing cancer.

Benefits of CBD

Most research, thus far, has centered in studies using animals or biopsied human tissue. In a study cited in a 2011 issue of *PLOS ONE,* researchers studied "biopsies from individuals with ulcerative colitis" and found that "CBD was an effective anti-inflammatory agent, whether the biopsy was from a patient in remission or experiencing active disease." The researchers found that CBD affects certain cells that are the first line of defense against harmful pathogens. Normally, these cells stimulate inflammation in the GI tract by manufacturing a certain protein, whereas CBD modulates its production, therefore reducing inflammation.

Research suggests that CBD offers relief from symptoms of ulcerative colitis, such as pain relief, reduces nausea, and stimulates the appetite. In an article published in the October 2011 edition of *European Journal of Gastroenterology & Hepatology,* the authors stated that cannabis is commonly used by IBD patients for symptom relief, in particular for those with a history of abdominal surgery and chronic abdominal pain.

How to Use

Recommended dosage is 3 to 30 mg of CBD taken twice daily. A combination of Raw CBDA extracts with gold concentrated extracts offer the widest possible range of cannabinoids in hemp. THC if tolerable may provide additional pain relief. Omega 3 ALA in addition to marine omega 3 EPA and DHA may enhance benefits. *See also* **CROHN'S DISEASE**

Resources

Unlike the resource centers for information on marijuana, resources for more information regarding CBD oil products are quite limited. Many of the CBD related websites are set up to sell products rather than focus on the research being conducted on hemp. We have tried to avoid including resources that sell CBD products. Please note all information below may be subject to change. It is therefore important to contact these centers before planning a visit.

CANNIBINOID THERAPY

CBD Resource Center

This resource center is a point of reference for recent studies, tests, or just general resources regarding CBD research and certain conditions.
https://blog.nectarleaf.com/ cbd-resource-center/
1-415-935-1424

HEMP OIL RESOURCE GUIDE

Healthy Hemp Oil LTD

A resource that provides basic information that one should know about using and buying canabidiol, including benefits, current research, legal status, and the history of cannabidiol.
Office 3 Unit R
Penfold Works
Imperial Way
Watford, Herts United Kingdom, WD24 4YY
https://healthyhempoil.com/ cannabidiol/
1-844-HEMPOIL (436-7645)

CBD Resource Center

This is a resource site that provides documentation, videos, and testimonials to help create a better understanding of CBD and how to use CBD products.

Soul Purpose

https://soulpurpose.com/cbd-resource-center

Project CBD

A website covering how CBD works, CBD dosing, and medical conditions that can benefit from CBD.
https://www.projectcbd.org/

CBD Oil Education

A website that includes common questions asked about CBD, the basics of CBD, and a product guide.
https://www.medicalmarijuanainc.com/cbd-oil-education

Medical News Today

Everything you need to know about CBD Oil: basics, benefits, risks and side effects and how to use CBD.
https://www.medicalnewstoday.com/articles/317221

Sona CBD

A website that provides an understanding of CBD and its powerful benefits.
https://sonacbd.com/cbd-resources/

Medical Jane

Medical Jane provides free medical cannabis education and resources to suffering patients. Provides a step-by-step patient guide to find optimal dosage and delivery method.
www.medicaljane.com/

About the Author

Earl Mindell, RPh, MH, PhD, is a registered pharmacist and college educator. He is also the award-winning author of over twenty best-selling books, including *Earl Mindell's New Vitamin Bible*. Dr. Mindell was inducted into the California Pharmacists Association's Hall of Fame in 2007, and was awarded the President's Citation for Exemplary Service from Bastyr University in 2012. He is on the Board of Directors of the California College of Natural Medicine and serves on the Dean's Professional Advisory Group, School of Pharmacy, Chapman University.

Index

A

Addiction, opiate, 25–27

ADHD, 27

Age-related macular degeneration (AMD), 28–30

Agonists, partial, 26

Alzheimer's disease, 30–33

AMD, 33

American Psychiatric Association, 51

Antagonists, 26

Antiemetics, 36

Anti-inflammatory drugs. *See also* NSAIDs. 38, 49–50, 73–74, 95

effects of CBD, 68, 81, 95

Antihistamines, 36, 76

Antipsychotics, 92–93

Anti-pyretic, 38

Anxiety disorders, 33–35

Appetite loss, 35–37

Arthritis, 37–39

Attention deficit hyperactivity disorder (ADHD), 40–42

Atopic dermatitis. *See* eczema.

B

Beta-amyloid, 33

Bioaccumulator, 15

Bioavailability, 9, 13, 14

Blood clots, 42–45

C

Cancer, 45–48

Cannabidiol (CBD)

extraction methods, 11–14

isolates, 13

oil, 3–11

products, 9–11

Cannabis, hemp plant, 14–15

Cannabis and Cannabinoid Research, 15–17

Cannabidiolic acid (CBDA), raw hemp extracts, 4–5

Cannafinoids/terpenes, benefits of, 21

Cardiovascular disease, 48

CBD, extracting methods

carbon dioxide method, 11–13

cold pressing, 11

nanotechnology delivery, 13–14

CBD oil, types

decarboxylated oil, 5–6

gold formula oil, 6–8

raw hemp oil, 4–5

CBD oil, what is it?, 3–4
CBD products
  balms, 9
  capsules /softgels, 8–9
  concentrates, 10
  drops/sprays, 9
  vaporizers, 10–11
  world of products, 13
Certificate of Analysis (COA), 9
Chemotherapy side effects, 48
Cholinesterase inhibitors. *See also* Alzheimer's disease.
Clinical endocannabinoid theory, 66
Colitis, 48
Corticosteroids, 49, 55, 74, 83, 95
Crohn's disease, 48–50

D
Delta-9-tetrahydracannabidiol. *See* THC.
Depression, 50–52
Dermatitis, atopc, 53–54
Drobainol (Marinol). *See* Synthetic cannabis drugs.

Eczema, 54–56
Epilepsy, 56–59
Eye disoroders, 59

F
Fibromyalgia, 60–62
FM, 62

G
Gabet, Dr. Yankel, 39

Glaucoma, 62–64
Gold formula hemp extracts, 6–8
GRAS (Generally Recognized as Safe), 7, 16

H
Headache, 64–66
Heart disease, 67–69
High blood pressure, 69–72

I
Inflammation, 72–75
Insomnia, 75–78
Irritable bowel syndrome (IBS), 78–81

J
Journal of Bone Health, 39

L
15-LOX, *See* Cannabidiolic acid.

M
Macular degeneration, 81
Memantine. *See also* Alzheimer's disease.
Migraine headache, 81
Multiple sclerosis (MS), 82–85
MS, 82

N
Nausea/ vomiting, 86–87
New England Journal of Medicine, 32

Nonsteroidal Anti-inflammatory Drugs (NSAIDs), 38, 73

O
Opiate addiction, 88
Opioid abuse, dependency, 27

P
Panic attack, 88
Potency, 18–20
PMS, 88
Phytocannabinoids, 5, 6
Post-traumatic stress disorder, 88
Premenstrual Dysphoric Disorder (PMDD). *See* Premenstrual syndrome.
Premenstrual syndrome (PMS), 88–91
PRISH, 73

R
Rheumatoid arthritis, 37, 38, 39, 72, 74

Rheumatology, 2013 study, 38–39
Russo, Dr. Ethan. *See* Clinical Endocannabinoid Theory.

S
Sativex, 84
Selective serotonin reuptake inhibitors (SSRIs), 34, 35, 52
Serotonin norepinephrine reuptake inhibitors (SNRIs), 34
Schizophrenia, 91–93
Schubert, Dr. David, study on cannabinoids for Alzheimer's, 33
Skin Conditions, 93
Sleep disorders, 93

T
Thrombosis, 93
Thyroid disorders, 94
Tumors, 45

U
Ulcerative colitis, 94, 96

Healing with Medical Marijuana

Getting Beyond the Smoke and Mirrors

Dr. Mark Sircus

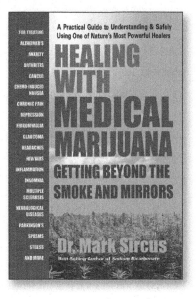

Imagine that there is an effective treatment for dozens of serious ailments—from cancer and Parkinson's disease to headaches and depression. Now imagine that the government is preventing you from using it because it is derived from a controversial herb. Cannabis, more commonly called marijuana, is still looked upon by many people as a social evil; yet, scientific evidence clearly shows that the compounds it contains can reduce, halt, and in many cases, reverse some of our most serious health conditions. In *Healing with Medical Marijuana,* best-selling author and medical researcher Dr. Mark Sircus has written a clear guide to understanding the power of the cannabis plant in combating numerous disorders

While more and more states are now legalizing medical marijuana as a safe and effective treatment method, the controversy continues to block its use for the majority of the population—in spite of the relief it can provide. For those who may be unable to obtain medical marijuana to treat their individual conditions, this book is designed to provide options that can offer the much-needed help they are seeking.

$16.95 US • 192 pages • 6 x 9-inch quality paperback • ISBN 978-0-7570-0441-4

What You Must Know About Allergy Relief

How to Overcome the Allergies
You Have & Find the Hidden
Allergies That Make You Sick

Earl Mindell, RPh, and
Pamela Wartian Smith, MD

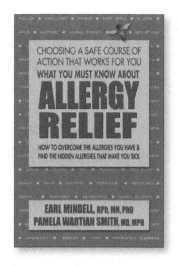

When most people have allergies, they
know it. Symptoms come quickly and
can range from mild reactions like
sneezing and itching to severe, often
debilitating effects like anaphylaxis.
Millions of others, however, suffer from allergies and don't even
know it. Allergies and intolerances are often the hidden culprits
that lie at the heart of a number of health conditions. If you are an
allergy sufferer or have a recurring health issue that you can't seem
to resolve, *What You Must Know About Allergy Relief* is the book
for you. Written by a pharmacist and medical doctor, it provides
important answers to the most common questions about allergies—
what causes them, how they can affect your health, and most
important, what you can do to overcome them.

Written in a clear, reader-friendly style, this book is divided into
three parts. Part One presents an overview of the causes of allergic
conditions as well as their most effective treatment methods—
both conventional and alternative. Part Two offers sound advice
and practical tips for dealing with asthma, skin conditions, and
other allergic reactions both at home and in the workplace. In Part
Three, the authors provide a comprehensive guide to anti-allergy
medications, supplements, and other treatment options.

Beautifully written, easy to understand, and up-to-date, *What You
Must Know About Allergy Relief* offers the tools to identify hidden
allergies as well as the means to relieve their symptoms.

$17.95 US • 288 pages • 6 x 9-inch quality paperback • ISBN 978-0-7570-0437-7

Your Blood Never Lies

How to Read a Blood Test for a Longer, Healthier Life

James B. LaValle, RPh, CCN

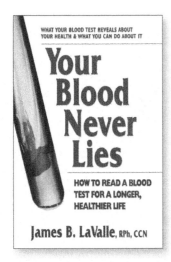

WHAT YOUR BLOOD TEST REVEALS ABOUT YOUR HEALTH & WHAT YOU CAN DO ABOUT IT

Your Blood Never Lies

HOW TO READ A BLOOD TEST FOR A LONGER, HEALTHIER LIFE

James B. LaValle, RPh, CCN

If you're like most people, you probably rely on your doctor to interpret the results of your blood tests, which contain a wealth of information on the state of your health. A blood test can tell you how well your kidneys and liver are functioning, your potential for heart disease and diabetes, the strength of your immune system, the chemical profile of your blood, and many other important facts about the state of your health. And yet, most of us cannot decipher these results ourselves, nor can we even formulate the right questions to ask about them—or we couldn't, until now.

In *Your Blood Never Lies,* best-selling author Dr. James LaValle clears the mystery surrounding blood test results. In simple language, he explains all the information found on a typical lab report—the medical terminology, the numbers and percentages, and the laboratory jargon—and makes it accessible. This means that you will be able to look at your own blood test results and understand the significance of each biological marker being measured.

To help you take charge of your health, Dr. LaValle also recommends the most effective standard and complementary treatments for dealing with any problematic findings. Rounding out the book are explanations of lab values that do not appear on the standard blood test, but that should be requested for a more complete picture of your current physiological condition.

Your Blood Never Lies provides the up-to-date information you need to understand your results and take control of your life.

$16.95 US • 368 pages • 6 x 9-inch quality paperback • ISBN 978-0-7570-0350-9

What You Must Know About Homeopathic Remedies

A Concise Guide to Understanding and Using Homeopathy

Earl Mindell, RPh, MH, PhD

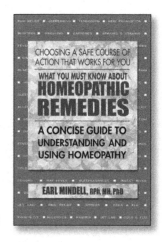

Go to any pharmacy today, and you'll find dozens of homeopathic products that provide relief from a host of health issues—from stress to sinus congestion to jet lag. The fact is, homeopathy has become a widely accepted way of treating many common emotional and physical disorders. In response to the growing interest in this traditional method of healing, best-selling author Dr. Earl Mindell has written a simple and concise guide to understanding and using homeopathic remedies.

$9.95 US • 96 pages • 6 x 9-inch quality paperback • ISBN 978-0-7570-0457-5

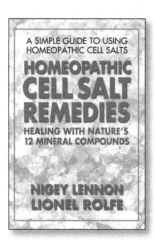

Homeopathic Cell Salt Remedies

Healing with Nature's 12 Mineral Compounds

Nigey Lennon and Lionel Rolfe

Homeopathic Cell Salt Remedies is a simple, comprehensive guide to healing with mineral compounds called cell salts. The book provides full descriptions of the twelve cell salts and discusses how they can be used to treat common conditions.

$12.95 US • 160 pages • 6 x 9-inch quality paperback • ISBN 978-0-7570-0250-2